ACCIDENT
and
EMERGENCY
medicine

A SURVIVAL GUIDE

ACCIDENT
and
EMERGENCY
medicine

A SURVIVAL GUIDE

Ashis Banerjee
MS FRCS (Ed) FRCS (Eng) DTM&H Consultant
Accident and Emergency Department
Whittington Hospital NHS Trust
LONDON

W.B. Saunders Company Ltd
LONDON PHILADELPHIA TORONTO SYDNEY TOKYO

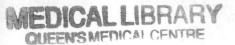
W. B. Saunders Company Ltd 24–28 Oval Road
London NWI 7DX

The Curtis Center
Independence Square West
Philadelphia, PA 19106-3399, USA

Harcourt Brace & Company
55 Horner Avenue
Toronto, Ontario M8Z 4X6, Canada

Harcourt Brace & Company, Australia
30–52 Smidmore Street
Marrickville, NSW 2204, Australia

Harcourt Brace & Company, Japan
Ichibancho Central Building, 22–1
Ichibancho, Chiyoda-ku,
Tokyo 102, Japan

A catalogue record for this book is available from
the British Library

ISBN 0–7020–2210–1   1000814490

Typeset by Florencetype Ltd, Stoodleigh, Devon
Printed in Great Britain by Mackays of Chatham plc,
Chatham, Kent

Contents

>

> Contents

>

> Contents

>

> Contents

>

> Contents

>

> Contents

Preface

The newly appointed Senior House Officer in Accident and Emergency has to acquire a large amount of information in the shortest possible time. He or she may encounter several conditions or situations for which there is no previous experience to draw upon. The demands of the job require rapid decisions to be taken on the background of increasing litigation for medical negligence. While the role of induction courses, structured teaching programmes and shop floor supervision by middle grade and senior staff is undeniable there is still the need for a portable source of useful basic information to which rapid reference can be made.

It is inevitable in a book of this size that totally comprehensive cover is not possible; the selection of topics is based on the commonly encountered situations in the average Accident and Emergency Department in the United Kingdom. Wherever available national guidelines have been adhered to. Management guidelines are not overtly prescriptive, taking into account local variations in medical practice.

I am grateful for all advice and suggestions made over the years by both junior and senior colleagues who are, however, too numerous to individually name. Any errors must remain my responsibility.

I sincerely hope that this book will be a useful adjunct to training for Senior House Officers.

A Banerjee

March 1996

1 General principles

Documentation

Accident and Emergency (A&E) records form part of the patient's permanent records and are of considerable medicolegal significance.

They must be concise, relevant and written legibly.

All notes must be timed, dated and signed legibly.

The high turnover of junior medical staff makes it imperative that the signature is identifiable. Where it is not, the doctor's names must be entered in block letters.

All notes must be made contemporaneously.

All positive findings and all relevant negative findings must be recorded.

Facetious and potentially libellous remarks must not be made in the notes.

Obscure abbreviations must be avoided.

All investigations ordered and their results where available must be noted in the record.

The ultimate disposal of the patient (e.g. discharged, referred for second opinion, admitted or died) must be entered.

For all referrals, the time of referral and the name, status and specialty of the doctor to whom the referral was made should be noted.

Communication with General Practitioners

General practitioners (GP) coordinate the overall care and follow-up of patients registered with them.

It is vitally important that the GP is notified of patients registered with them who attend the A&E department.

The mechanism whereby this is done may vary from department to department, e.g. handwritten letter, computer generated letter, photocopy of A&E record, tear-off copy of A&E records. If a situation requires urgent communication, the use of the telephone is recommended. Occasionally, the GP is able to provide useful information regarding past medical history and current medication.

The GP always needs to be notified of:

1. A&E attendance
2. Investigations done in A&E and their results
3. Final diagnosis or differential diagnosis
4. Follow-up arrangements made in hospital
5. Any follow-up action that may be needed in the community
6. Any new treatment instituted or any alterations to previous treatment (including dosage and duration where appropriate)
7. Any results that are not immediately available (e.g. culture reports) should be directed to the GP by recording this fact on the requisition form
8. Death of a patient registered with them

Police Statements

Writing police statements is a statutory duty of A&E doctors, particularly in the course of treating assault victims.

The income earned from such statements is classified as Category 2 (NHS Act) work and is taxable.

The statement must begin with an identification of the doctor by name, qualifications and designation, and then of the victim by name and date of birth.

Only facts pertaining to the injuries sustained must be given, and not opinions.

Details of alleged assault should not be recorded as these are hearsay evidence.

Standard forms must be used.

All entries must be signed and countersigned by a colleague.

A photocopy must be kept of all completed statements for future reference.

The fee note must be completed. It is better to give a home or permanent address for purposes of receiving the fee and for further contact, as this may occur after the doctor has left the A&E department.

Non-medical terms must be used wherever possible. Diagrams are useful.

No police statement should be provided without written consent from the individual on whom the report is being compiled.

Inter-Hospital Referrals

Should ideally be coordinated by a middle-grade or senior member of A&E for critically ill patients.

PRIOR TO TRANSFER

Ensure airway patency is maintained and that haemo-dynamic status is stable, with bleeding having been controlled

TRANSFER

Ensure adequate personnel accompany the patient, usually a nurse and anaesthetist

Monitoring should be continued en route: blood pressure and heart rate, electrocardiogram (ECG), pulse oximetry (battery powered, with an adequate life)

SEND WITH PATIENT

Photocopy of all hospital notes
X-rays
Results of investigations
Labelled blood samples if available
An additional handwritten letter may be needed

Major Incident Policy

Every junior doctor working in an A&E department should be aware of the existence and location of the departmental major policy document and must have read the section relevant to his or herself (often in the form of an action card).

The basic components of a major incident are:

Activation: usually by the ambulance service

Call-out procedure: organized for the hospital by the switchboard. This may involve:

Group paging of key personnel

Use of cascades of sequential communication by the hospital personnel initially activated

Use of tannoy system or other public address facility within the hospital

Designated staff functions: in the form of action cards

Allocated areas for specific functions:

- Reception
- Triage
- Walking wounded area
- Stretcher case area
- Control room
- Press liaison office

Debriefing and **counselling** after the incident is called down and the victims have been adequately dealt with

2 Cardiovascular emergencies

Cardiac Arrest

This is essentially a clinical diagnosis made in the following circumstances:

- Sudden collapse
- Loss of consciousness
- Absent central pulse (e.g. carotid or femoral)

No time must be wasted
  Checking pupillary light reactions
  Listening for heart sounds

The **sequence of action** includes:
  Note time and call for help. This usually means activation of the cardiac arrest team

BASIC LIFE SUPPORT is initiated:

Clear **airway** of blood, vomit, food or dentures
  Position to open airway
    Backward tilt of head
    Support chin
    Jaw thrust

Check **breathing**

If no spontaneous breathing
  Give two breaths of expired air ventilation (mouth to mouth)

If thereafter no spontaneous breathing
  Check carotid pulse

If no palpable pulse
  Commence external cardiac massage
    Place heel of one hand over lower sternum and heel of the other hand over the first with fingers interlocked
    Keep elbows locked in extension
    Depress sternum by 1–2 inches

Synchronize compressions with ventilation
  For one rescuer: 80 compressions/minute
                    15 compressions to 2 ventilations
  For two rescuers: 60 compressions/minute
                    5 compressions to 1 ventilation   >

> Cardiac Arrest

This usually progresses to **ADVANCED LIFE SUPPORT**

Ventilation
Oropharyngeal airway + self-inflating bag/valve device
Orotracheal intubation with cuffed endotracheal tube

Circulation
Continue cardiac massage
Obtain central venous access if necessary

Connect the patient to the ECG monitor to determine the rhythm and treat accordingly (Figs 1–5)

Periodically monitor effectiveness of cardiopulmonary resuscitation (CPR):
Is a central pulse palpable with cardiac massage?
Are both lungs expanding equally with ventilation?
Are the pupils symmetrical and reacting to light?

In hospital, arrests are often **witnessed**. In these circumstances, ventricular fibrillation is highly likely. The above programme may be modified to include:
A precordial thump
Defibrillation with an unsynchronized 200 J shock

In general, if fibrillation is likely, the ABC sequence (**A**ir, **B**reathing, **C**irculation) may be initially dispensed with in favour of defibrillation, which is often all that is necessary.

DECISIONS TO TERMINATE CPR depend on several factors:

- Underlying disease (e.g. terminal malignancy)
- Duration of CPR and response thereto
- Core temperature if hypothermic

In the hospital situation it is usual to proceed rapidly to advanced life support.

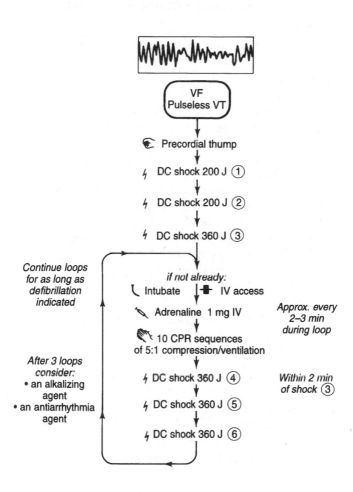

Fig. 1 Ventricular fibrillation (VF).

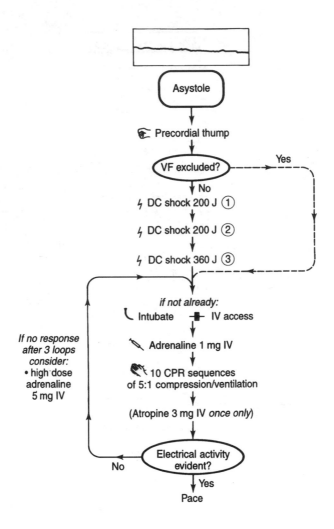

Fig. 2. Asystole.

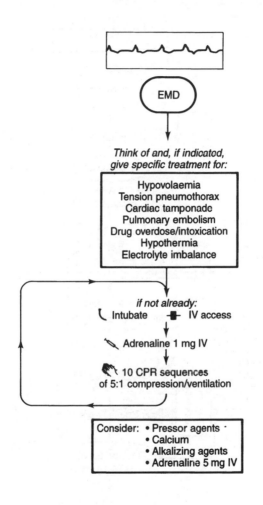

Fig. 3 Electromechanical dissociation (EMD).

Cardiopulmonary Resuscitation

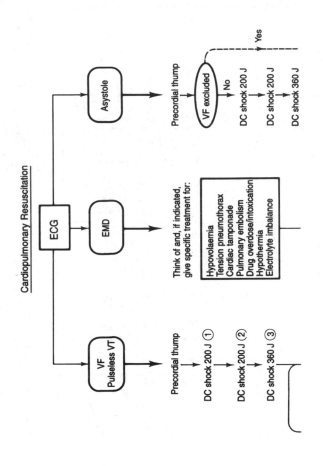

ECG

VF Pulseless VT | **EMD** | **Asystole**

Precordial thump
DC shock 200 J ①
DC shock 200 J ②
DC shock 360 J ③

Think of and, if indicated, give specific treatment for:

Hypovolaemia
Tension pneumothorax
Cardiac tamponade
Pulmonary embolism
Drug overdose/intoxication
Hypothermia
Electrolyte imbalance

Precordial thump
VF excluded
Yes
No
DC shock 200 J
DC shock 200 J
DC shock 360 J

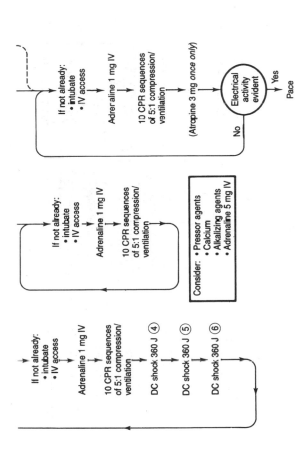

Fig. 4 Summary of cardiopulmonary resuscitation. Redrawn from *Resuscitation*, 24, Guidelines for Advanced Life Support, 111–121, 1992 with kind permission from Elsevier Science Ireland Ltd, Co. Clare, Ireland.

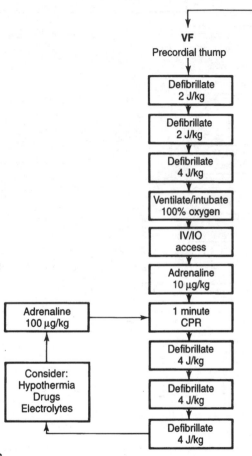

VF

Precordial thump

Defibrillate
2 J/kg

Defibrillate
2 J/kg

Defibrillate
4 J/kg

Ventilate/intubate
100% oxygen

IV/IO
access

Adrenaline
10 µg/kg

Adrenaline
100 µg/kg

1 minute
CPR

Consider:
Hypothermia
Drugs
Electrolytes

Defibrillate
4 J/kg

Defibrillate
4 J/kg

Defibrillate
4 J/kg

NOTES
1. ETT adrenaline dose ×10 if IV/IO not established within 90 seconds
2. After 3 loops, consider alkalizing and/or antiarrhythmic agents

PAEDIATRIC ADVANCED LIFE SUPPORT

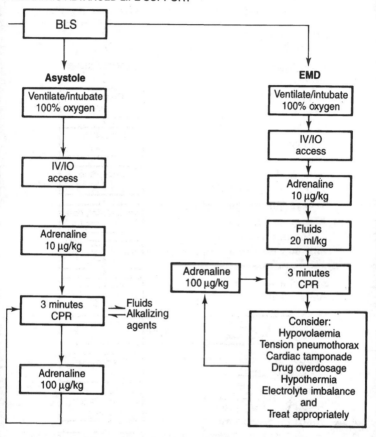

NOTE
ETT adrenaline dose ×10 if IV/IO not established within 90 seconds

Fig. 5 Paediatric advanced life support. Redrawn from *Resuscitation*, 24, Guidelines for Advanced Life Support, 111–121, 1992 with kind permission from Elsevier Science Ireland Ltd, Co. Clare, Ireland.

Acute Chest Pain

History taking is of vital importance in assessment of chest pain, allowing recognition of the following patterns:

Cardiac ischaemic
 Pressing, crushing, constricting retrosternal pain
 May radiate to left arm, neck, and jaws
 Associated with sweating
 Unaffected by movement or deep inspiration

Aortic
 Sudden onset of severe tearing anterior chest pain, maximal from the onset
 Radiation to the back

Pericardial
 Stabbing retrosternal or epigastric pain
 May radiate to left shoulder and neck
 Aggravated by movement of upper torso and by deep breathing
 Relieved by sitting upright and leaning forward

Oesophageal reflux
 Retrosternal burning pain
 Worse with recumbency
 Relieved by antacids
 Waterbrash

Pleuritic
 Sharp pain increased by deep breathing and movements

Musculoskeletal
 Insidious onset often
 Sharp localized pain
 Increased by position change, deep breathing and shoulder girdle movements

Neurological
 Dermatomal pain followed by vesicular skin rash

> Acute Chest Pain

A history of **cardiovascular risk factors** must be sought if ischaemic cardiac pain is suspected. Also obtain a history of pre-existing ischaemic heart disease.

CLINICAL EXAMINATION is often non-contributory and initial management is usually dictated by the history. Specific features to be looked for include:

- Signs of **sympathetic activation**
    Pallor
    Sweating
    Tachycardia
- Chest wall tenderness that exactly reproduces the pain
- Chest signs
    Pleural rubs
    Asymmetric chest expansion
    Asymmetric breath sounds
    Localized crepitations/bronchial breathing

Specific **INVESTIGATIONS** include:

- 12-lead ECG
- Chest X-ray
- Serum cardiac enzymes
    Rapid assay of creatine kinase (CK)-MB

CARDIOVASCULAR RISK FACTORS

Major
    Hypertension
    Hypercholesterolaemia
    Smoking
    Diabetes mellitus

Minor
    Obesity
    Physical inactivity
    Stress

ECG Interpretation

A systematic approach is necessary to obtain maximal information. A 12-lead ECG is mandatory in analysing acute cardiac conditions.

The following sequence is recommended:

Check **name** of patient
      date and **time** of recording

Do not rely unduly on diagnostic printouts which can be inaccurate and are susceptible to artefact

Rhythm
Regular or irregular
Note intervals between successive R waves

Rate
Count number of large squares (5 mm) between two successive R waves and divide into 300

or

Count number of QRS complexes in 3 seconds (15 large squares) and multiply by 20

Axis
Leads I, aVF, II
Mean QRS axis: −30 to +110°

P Waves
Presence/absence
Shape
Duration: < 0.08 seconds (two small squares)
Height: < 2.5 mm

P–R Interval
Duration less than one large square (five small squares), i.e. < 0.20 seconds

Q Waves

QRS Complexes
Duration less than three small squares (0.12 seconds)
Total amplitude in any one lead < 35 mm

T Waves

ST Segment
Normally isoelectric

>

> ECG Interpretation

QT Interval

Less than two small squares (0.40 seconds)

The above measurements assume paper calibration at a speed of 25 mm per square

Each small square = 1 mm

= 0.04 seconds

= 40 milliseconds

Each large square = 5 mm

= 0.20 seconds

= 20 milliseconds

1 mV produces a vertical deflection of 10 mm (two large squares)

Each fifth line is heavier to facilitate counting

When analysing an arrhythmia, the following questions need to be asked:

Is atrial activity present?

Are P waves seen (usually best seen in inferior leads II, III, aVF or right precordial leads)

Is the QRS complex
normal or wide?
fast or slow?
regular or irregular?

Is there any relation between P waves and QRS complexes?

Are there any premature beats or any abnormal pauses?

Palpitations

This is defined as an unpleasant awareness of the heart's action. It is usually due to an increased heart rate, but can be caused by missed beats or slow rhythms.

The basic assessment of the patient with palpitations who is found to have tachycardia (heart rate over 120 beats per minute) should include:

- Assessment of haemodynamic status
     Level of consciousness
     Peripheral perfusion
     Blood pressure
- Evidence of overt or covert blood loss
- Current medications
- **Venous blood**:
     Urea and electrolytes (U&E)
- A 12-lead ECG, which should allow categorization as follows:

Narrow QRS complexes: < 0.12 seconds
  Regular rate
     Sinus tachycardia
     Atrial tachycardia
     Junctional tachycardia
  Irregular rate
     Atrial fibrillation
     Atrial flutter/tachycardia with variable AV conduction

Broad QRS complexes: > 0.14 seconds
  Regular rate
     Ventricular tachycardia
     Supraventricular tachycardia with aberrant intraventricular conduction or with pre-existing bundle branch block
  Irregular rate
     Atrial fibrillation with aberrant or pre-excited conduction to the ventricles

Diagnosis of Broad Complex Tachycardia

The haemodynamic status is of no value. Many patients with ventricular tachycardia are haemodynamically stable when first seen.

USEFUL FEATURES

Pre-existing coronary artery disease or myocardial disease (favours VT)

Independent atrial activity (excludes SVT)

Demonstrable P waves

Ventriculoatrial dissociation

Capture beats

Fusion beats

Carotid sinus massage

May terminate SVT

QRS complex

Duration > 0.14 seconds: VT

Axis: left axis deviation

Morphology

RBBB pattern: SVT

LBBB pattern: VT

Concordance

All QRS complexes in precordial leads V1–V6 either upright or inverted: VT

MANAGEMENT

Always identify the underlying rhythm on the basis of the 12-lead ECG

Obtain venous access

If haemodynamically stable, do not give blind pharmacological treatment if you are unsure of the mechanism of the tachyarrhythmia

If haemodynamically unstable, refer urgently to the medical on-call team and notify an anaesthetist, as DC cardioversion will be required

>

ADENOSINE

This is a valuable drug for treating arrhythmias in the A&E department

It will terminate supraventricular tachycardia originating in the atrioventricular node and produce transient atrioventricular nodal block in arrhythmias originating in the atria

It can be used as a diagnostic agent in broad or narrow complex regular tachycardia of uncertain cause. It will not terminate ventricular arrhythmias

It is given as a rapid bolus into a peripheral vein and followed by a saline flush

The initial dose of 3 mg in adults may be followed by further doses of 6 mg and then 12 mg at 1 to 2 minute intervals if needed

For children the initial dose of 0.05 mg/kg increases by 0.05 mg/kg increments to a maximum bolus dose of 0.25 mg/kg

DEFINITIVE MANAGEMENT OF VENTRICULAR TACHYCARDIA

Intravenous **lignocaine** 2 mg/kg over 5 minutes

If the patient is hypotensive or if lignocaine fails,
DC cardioversion is indicated

Medical referral is always needed

Syncope

Syncope can be defined as a transient loss of consciousness and loss of postural tone, followed by complete recovery, and is due to global reduction of cerebral blood flow. To the onlooker it is often a dramatic situation leading to the individual being brought to an A&E department, particularly if the episode occurred in a public place.

The diagnosis is made usually on the basis of the history, aided by clinical examination.

HISTORY taking should elucidate the following points:

- Precipitating factors, e.g. emotion, pain, prolonged standing, neck movement, micturition, cough
- Warning symptoms
- Previous episodes of a similar nature
- Past medical history
- Current medications

A reliable eye witness account is crucial. Specific questioning is directed toward:

> Post-episode recovery, e.g. was drowsiness or confusion a feature (more suggestive of a postictal situation)
>
> Any seizure activity during the episode: occasional clonic jerks of the limbs may be associated with any more prolonged episode of syncope

ASSESSMENT includes:

- Level of consciousness
- Vital signs:
  > Pulse rate
  > Supine and standing blood pressure (BP)
  >> Systolic fall of 20 mmHg or more after 3 minutes standing indicates significant postural hypotension
  > Blood pressure in both upper limbs
- Signs of injury secondary to falling
- Auscultation of the heart for murmurs
- 12-lead ECG
- Carotid sinus massage with ECG monitoring (if no carotid bruit) if carotid sinus syndrome suspected   >

> Syncope

The common **CAUSES** of syncope are:

Situational
Vasovagal attack (simple faint), which occurs in response
 to an identifiable noxious stimulus or to prolonged
 standing
Micturition, cough or defaecation syncope

Postural hypotension
Drugs
Autonomic insufficiency
Peripheral neuropathy

Cardiogenic
Bradycardia
 Complete atrioventricular block (Stokes-Adams attacks)
Tachyarrhythmia
 Supraventricular tachycardia
 Ventricular tachycardia
Low fixed cardiac output
 Aortic stenosis

Hypovolaemia

Carotid sinus syncope

Further **INVESTIGATION** (including 12-lead ECG and
Holter monitoring) is indicated for:

- Effort-induced syncope
- Inappropriate syncope
   No warning
   No precipitant
- Syncope associated with cardiac symptoms
   Especially palpitations

Where a diagnosis of vasovagal syncope is made, the
patient can be reassured and discharged from hospital.

Acute Myocardial Infarction

TYPICAL PRESENTATION

Central chest pain of crushing, pressing or constricting character lasting longer than 30 minutes. Often radiates to the neck, jaws, shoulder and arm. Associated sympathetic overactivity is often present, with sweating and tachycardia.

ATYPICAL PRESENTATIONS

These are more frequent in the elderly

- Sudden onset of shortness of breath (acute left ventricular failure)
- Atypical location of pain (arms, back, jaws)
- Exacerbation of pre-existing heart failure
- 'Indigestion'
- Nausea and vomiting only
- Profound fatigue
- Embolic phenomena: peripheral (limb ischaemia or gangrene) or cerebral (stroke) emboli
- Syncope
- Acute onset of dysrhythmia with palpitations
- Acute confusion

The **DEFINITIVE DIAGNOSIS** in the A&E department is usually made on the basis of the initial 12-lead ECG or on the development of typical changes on serial 12-lead ECGs. A normal initial ECG does not exclude the diagnosis.

Referral must be on clinical grounds. In all patients attending with the above symptoms a specific note must be made of **cardiovascular risk factors**, which adds ammunition to the diagnosis of myocardial infarction.

The typical ECG changes evolve as follows:

Hyperacute
Elevated ST segment
Tall wide T wave

Fully evolved acute
Pathological Q wave
Deep: more than one-third of height of R wave   >

> Acute Myocardial Infarction

> Wide: more than one little square (0.04 seconds or more)

Elevated ST segment

Inverted T wave

Reciprocal ST depression

Loss of R wave amplitude

Other ECG **patterns** of myocardial infarction include:

ST segment depression with T wave inversion (sub-endocardial infarction)

Tall, wide R waves with ST segment depression in V1 and V2

PHYSICAL EXAMINATION is usually of limited value in the diagnosis. The following may be observed:

- Pallor, sweating, anxiety
- Fourth heart sound
- Basal lung crepitations
- The syndrome of right ventricular infarction
  Hypotension
  Raised jugular venous pressure
  Clear lung fields
  Tricuspid regurgitation
- In later stages:
  Pericardial friction rubs
  Systolic murmurs (VSD or acute mitral incompetence)

Localization of the infarct is possible by determining the leads in which the typical changes occur:

- Extensive anterior
  I, II, aVL, V1–V6
- Anteroseptal
  I, aVL, V2–V4
- Anterolateral
  I, aVL, V4–V6
- Inferior
  aVF, II, III

Once the diagnosis of acute myocardial infarction is suspected or proven: >

> Acute Myocardial Infarction

- Establish venous access
- Administer 60% oxygen by face mask
- Relieve pain
  Slow intravenous injection of an opiate, e.g. diamorphine 5 mg at 1 mg/minute
- Administer an antiemetic
  Intravenous metoclopramide 10 mg or cyclizine 25–50 mg
- Commence ECG monitoring
- Give aspirin 150–300 mg in the absence of known hypersensitivity
- Commence thrombolysis where indicated

If the diagnosis is not proven, sending venous blood for rapid assay for CK-MB, if at least 3 hours have elapsed since the onset of pain, may be helpful.

THROMBOLYSIS

Absolute contraindications

Aortic dissection
Head injury or cerebrovascular accident (CVA) within past 6 weeks
Neurosurgery within past 2 months
Gastrointestinal bleeding
Intracranial aneurysm or neoplasm

Relative contraindications

Major surgery, obstetric delivery or organ biopsy in past 10 days
Past history of gastrointestinal bleeding
Severe arterial hypertension (systolic BP over 200 mmHg or diastolic BP over 110 mmHg)
Bleeding diathesis
Major trauma
Diabetic haemorrhagic or proliferative retinopathy

Unstable Angina

This is a clinical diagnosis, made in the following circumstances:

● Angina at rest
● Exertional angina with pain provoked by minimal exertion or stress
● Abrupt worsening of previously stable angina
● Recent onset of effort angina

The initial **MANAGEMENT** includes:

12-lead ECG
Intravenous access
Provision of pain relief
Adminstration of aspirin 150–300 mg
Medical referral is indicated as there is a risk of sudden
  death and of myocardial infarction
Triple therapy (oral beta blockers, intravenous nitrates and
  oral calcium antagonists) is required along with intensive monitoring
Some cardiologists also recommend heparin

Acute Left Ventricular Failure

This is a common condition in A&E practice. The usual presentation is with:

- Acute shortness of breath
- Orthopnoea
- Paroxysmal nocturnal dyspnoea
- Expectoration of frothy blood-stained sputum
- Bilateral basal crepitations and wheezing in the lungs

The usual **CAUSES** are:

Pump failure from myocardial disease
  Ischaemic heart disease
Pressure overload
  Systemic hypertension
  Aortic stenosis
Volume overload
  Aortic incompetence
  Mitral incompetence

Initial **ASSESSMENT** includes:

- Colour
- Ability to speak
- Vital signs
- Pulse oximetry
- Portable chest X-ray
- 12-lead ECG

CHEST X-RAY FINDINGS include:

Pulmonary venous congestion with distended upper lobe veins

Interstitial oedema leading to a hilar and/or perihilar haze, and to Kerley A and B lines

Alveolar oedema leading to fluffy bilaterally symmetrical infiltrates

MANAGEMENT includes:

Nursing **propped up**
High flow **oxygen** (60%) by mask
Venous access   >

> Acute Left Ventricular Failure

Opioids
  Diamorphine 2.5–5 mg intravenously or morphine 5–10
    mg intravenously

Diuretics
  Frusemide 40–80 mg intravenously

Vasodilators
  Glyceryl trinitrate infusion or sublingual glyceryl
    trinitrate

Inotropes if hypotensive
  Dopamine infusion
    5–20 µg/kg/minute
  or **Dobutamine** infusion
    5–20 µg/kg/minute

Referral to the on-call medical team

Pulmonary Embolism

Several different syndromes can lead to A&E department attendance:

1. Acute minor pulmonary embolism with pulmonary infarct
   Cough
   Pleuritic chest pain
   Haemoptysis
   Pleural friction rub
2. Acute massive pulmonary embolism
   Cardiovascular collapse from acute decrease in cardiac output
   Acute right ventricular failure
   Raised central venous pressure (CVP)
   Diastolic gallop rhythm
   Acute disturbance of pulmonary ventilation/perfusion, causing:
   Acute shortness of breath
   Arterial hypoxia (detectable on arterial blood gases (ABGs))
3. Subacute massive pulmonary embolism
   Pleuritic chest pain
   Insidious onset of shortness of breath
   Haemoptysis
   Right ventricular failure
4. Multiple pulmonary emboli
   Unexplained shortness of breath
   Unexplained tachypnoea

The **DIAGNOSIS** is aided by a combination of:

Symptoms at presentation
Identification of **risk factors** for **thromboembolic disease**
Physical signs
12-lead ECG, which may show rare but highly suggestive patterns, e.g.
Prominent S1 and Q3 and inverted T3
Right axis deviation

>

> Pulmonary Embolism

Transient right bundle branch block
rSR' or RSR' pattern
Right ventricular strain pattern
P pulmonale (tall P waves in II, III, aVF)
Arterial blood gases
Chest X-ray
Normal
or
Pulmonary infiltrate (pleural-based wedge-shaped
density)
Small pleural effusion
Focal oligaemia

A convincing presentation warrants **medical referral**.
Definitive diagnosis requires pulmonary ventilation/perfusion scanning and pulmonary angiography.

Hypertensive Emergencies

TYPES

Hypertensive encephalopathy
  Confusion
  Seizures
  Coma
  Malignant hypertension
    Retinal haemorrhages and exudates
Intracerebral haemorrhage
Aortic dissection
Phaeochromocytoma crisis
Eclampsia

ASSESSMENT

- History of hypertension
- Use of pressor agents
  Sympathomimetics
- Symptoms of cerebral, cardiac and visual dysfunction

EXAMINATION

- Blood pressure
- Optic fundi
- Neurological status
- Cardiopulmonary status
- Peripheral pulses
- Urinalysis dipstick testing

MANAGEMENT

Cautious acute reduction of blood pressure
Oral
  Nifedipine 5–10 mg sublingual
  or
  Atenolol 50–100 mg
Intravenous
  Labetalol 1–2 mg over 10 minutes
  Nitroprusside infusion titrated against continuously
    monitored blood pressure

Acute Dissection of the Thoracic Aorta

This condition has a high mortality if not promptly recognized.

The usual **presenting feature** is with pain, which may be retrosternal, interscapular or epigastric. The pain is tearing in quality, severe and maximal at the onset.

The associated features may include:
  Shock with raised systolic blood pressure
  Aortic branch occlusion in varying combinations
    Lower limb ischaemia
    Cerebrovascular accident
    Upper limb ischaemia
    Intestinal ischaemia
    Renal failure
    Paraplegia

The **predisposing features** include:
- Pregnancy
- Marfan's syndrome
- Coarctation of the aorta
- Polycystic kidneys

Initial **INVESTIGATION** in A&E includes:

12-lead ECG
Chest X-ray
  Superior mediastinal widening

Definitive diagnosis requires specialized imaging techniques:
- **CT scan**
- Aortography
- MRI scan
- Transoesophageal echocardiography

Referral to a cardiothoracic surgical unit is necessary.

Leaking Abdominal Aortic Aneurysm

This is a common cause of sudden death in the middle-aged and elderly.

Diagnosis is not always straightforward so a high index of clinical suspicion is needed.

The typical **PRESENTATION** is with:

- Sudden-onset severe abdominal and/or back pain
- Signs of shock
- Pulsatile abdominal mass. This may not always be easy to feel owing to hypotension, obesity or tamponade of pulsations

ATYPICAL PRESENTATIONS can occur, especially:

- Ureteric colic-like pain
- Syncope
- Unexplained high output cardiac failure (aortocaval fistula)
- Massive gastrointestinal bleeding (aortoenteric fistula)
- Peripheral ischaemia of the lower limbs
- Severe back pain alone

Where the diagnosis is made:

> The time spent in the A&E department should be minimized
>
> Immediately notify the duty surgeon, anaesthetist and the operating theatres
>
> Insert large-bore (14 gauge) cannulae in both upper extremities
>
> Obtain venous blood for full blood count (FBC), U&E, grouping and cross-matching of 10 units
>
> 12-lead ECG to exclude coexisting myocardial infarction
>
> Rapid transfer to operating room (OR)
>
> Later in the OR, CVP and arterial lines and urethral catheters are inserted

Where the diagnosis is uncertain and the patient is haemodynamically stable, surgical referral is warranted. Ultrasonography in the A&E department may help delineate the aneurysm.

Acute Lower Limb Ischaemia

This typically presents with a sudden onset of severe persistent lower limb pain, associated with numbness, paraesthesiae and loss of power in one or both lower limbs.

The signs of acute ischaemia that must be sought include:
    A pale cold limb
    Poor capillary return, as evidenced by delayed recovery from blanching on nail bed pressure
    Absent peripheral pulses
    Peripheral pulses undetectable by hand-held Doppler
    Loss of sensation in stocking fashion

The opposite lower limb must always be examined

The abdomen, groin and popliteal region must be palpated for evidence of arterial aneurysm

Acute ischaemia may be superimposed on a background of critical ischaemia, as evidenced by:
    Rest pain
    Impaired wound healing, with failure of trivial injuries to heal
    Patchy skin necrosis
    Ischaemic ulcers

Specific points to be noted in the **HISTORY** include:

- Previous arterial embolism
- Symptoms of peripheral arterial disease
    Intermittent claudication
- Recent myocardial infarction
- Atrial fibrillation

INITIAL MANAGEMENT includes:

Documentation of **vital signs**
Examination of all other peripheral pulses and of the heart
Provision of analgesia, e.g. papaveretum 15–20 mg intramuscularly
Venous access
Venous blood: FBC, U&E

>

> Acute Lower Limb Ischaemia

12-lead ECG
Surgical referral

Signs at presentation suggesting loss of limb viability:

- Fixed skin staining
- Gross muscle swelling
- Fixed plantarflexion of the ankle

Presence of these signs must not delay surgical referral

3 Respiratory emergencies

Chest X-Ray Analysis

Chest X-rays are often requested in A&E departments. Systematic assessment is necessary to obtain the maximum amount of available information and to avoid errors of omission.

ASSESSMENT of a chest film follows the following sequence:

1. Check that this is the film requested. In a department with a large number of patients and X-rays thereof, the wrong X-ray may be looked at
   Name of patient
   Date of X-ray
2. Check labelling of sides (right/left)
3. Ensure the technical quality of the film is adequate
   Centring
   The spinous processes of the vertebrae should be midway between the medial ends of the clavicles
   Degree of penetration
   Look at the visibility of the vertebral bodies, intervertebral discs and the tracheal bifurcation
   Whether taken in **full inspiration**
   The right dome of the diaphragm should be lower than the lower border of the anterior portion of the right 5th rib
4. Look at the **bones**
   Clavicles
   Ribs
   Scapulae
   Vertebrae
5. Look at the **soft tissues of the chest wall**
   Breast shadows
   Calcification
   Free air
6. Look at the **heart shadow**
   Size: note **cardiothoracic ratio**
   Maximum transverse diameter of the heart
   Maximum diameter of the chest

>

Shape
Retrocardiac shadows
 Left lower lobe collapse
 Mediastinal mass
 Hiatus hernia
7. Look at the **diaphragm**
 Level
 Shape
 Costophrenic angles
8. Look at the **trachea** and **mediastinum**
9. Look at the **lung fields**
 The lung fields are divided into three zones (upper, middle and lower) which are demarcated by the anterior ends of the 2nd and 4th ribs

PORTABLE A/P FILMS are often obtained in the emergency situation. The features of such films include:

- Labelling as anteroposterior (A/P)
- The medial scapulae are superimposed on the lung fields
- The clavicles are projected above the lung apices
- The heart and mediastinum appear magnified
- The ribs are more horizontal than usual

LATERAL FILMS of the chest may be needed to:

Localize lesions visible in posteroanterior (P/A) or A/P films
Visualize lesions in the retrosternal or retrocardiac space
Visualize lesions of the dorsal spine

The **CARDIAC SILHOUETTE** comprises the following structures:

Right border
 Superior vena cava
 Right pulmonary artery
 Right atrium
Left border
 Left superior vena cava/subclavian artery

>

> Chest X-Ray Analysis

Aortic knuckle
Left pulmonary artery
Left atrium
Left ventricle

Acute Shortness of Breath

Assessment of the acutely dyspnoeic patient includes:

ESTIMATION OF THE SEVERITY OF THE PRESENTING EPISODE

Level of consciousness
Ability to converse
Vital signs: respiratory rate, pulse rate, blood pressure
Use of accessory muscles of respiration
Evidence of suprasternal, intercostal and subcostal recession
Skin colour
Pulse oximetry
Is the episode **acute** or **acute on chronic**?
  Is there pre-existing cardiac or respiratory disease, with similar episodes in the past

What are the **ASSOCIATED SYMPTOMS**, which helps in elucidation of the likely cause:

1. **Pleuritic chest pain**
   Spontaneous pneumothorax
   Pulmonary embolism with infarction
   Pneumonia
   Rib fracture (spontaneous or following vigorous cough)
2. **Central non-pleuritic chest pain**
   Myocardial infarction with acute left ventricular failure
   Massive pulmonary embolism
3. **Cough and wheeze**
   Acute asthma
   Acute left ventricular failure ('cardiac asthma')
   Pneumonia
4. **No chest pain, cough or wheeze**
   Pulmonary embolism
   Tension pneumothorax
   Hypovolaemic shock
   Metabolic acidosis with respiratory compensation
5. **Stridor**
   Upper airway obstruction

>

CARBON DIOXIDE RETENTION

In severe shortness of breath from whatever cause, carbon dioxide retention ensues, producing the following:

- Peripheral vasodilatation
- Bounding peripheral pulses
- Coarse flapping tremor of outstretched hands
- Confusion
- Progressive drowsiness leading to coma
- Papilloedema

These are indicators of the need for urgent intervention, including anaesthetic assistance.

Important points in **HISTORY** taking, which may not be elicitable at the onset, include:

Mode of onset
Duration of symptoms
Progression of symptoms
Exercise tolerance in relation to activities of daily living
    Walking
    Climbing stairs
    Dressing, washing

Associated Symptoms

Cough
Sputum production
Haemoptysis
Chest pain
    Pleuritic
    Cardiac
Sleep disturbance due to:
    Orthopnea
    Paroxysmal nocturnal dyspnoea
Smoking history
Past history of cardiac, respiratory or allergic disorders
Occupation
    Exposure to dust, pollen, animals, chemicals   >

> Acute Shortness of Breath

INVESTIGATIONS

Venous blood: FBC and U&E

Arterial blood: ABGs (always state whether on room air or on oxygen and, if so, on what percentage)

Chest X-ray

12-lead ECG

Acute Asthma

Asthma can kill. Inadequate assessment and treatment are contributory factors.

Initial **ASSESSMENT** includes:

Assessment of the **severity of the current episode**, which is achieved from the following parameters:

- Level of consciousness
- Ability to speak
- Pulse rate, respiratory rate
- Peak expiratory flow rate (predicted value)
- Use of accessory muscles of respiration
- Arterial blood gases
- Tissue hypoxaemia on pulse oximetry
- Pulsus paradoxus (no longer used)

This allows identification of the following categories:

Life-threatening
    Exhaustion
    Silent chest
    Cyanosis
    Bradycardia
    Peak expiratory flow (PEF) less than 33% predicted or best
    Hypotension

Acute severe
    Unable to complete sentences in one breath
    Pulse rate > 110/minute
    Rising pulse rate
    Respiratory rate > 25/minute
    PEF 50% predicted or best

Arterial blood gas markers of severity
    Severe hypoxia pao_2 < 8 kPa (60 mmHg)
    Normal (5–6 kPa, 36–45 mmHg) or high $paco_2$
    Low pH

Assessment of the **severity of the underlying disease**:

- Past hospitalizations

>

> Acute Asthma

- Use of steroids
- Need for assisted ventilation

On arrival in the A&E department, all asthmatics who are short of breath receive a rapid assessment of:

- Colour
- Ability to speak
- Vital signs (blood pressure, pulse rate, respiratory rate)
- Peak flow
- Pulse oximetry

High flow **oxygen** (60%) is commenced by face mask
Nebulized **beta agonist** therapy is started
> Salbutamol 5 mg or terbutaline 10 mg, diluted in 5 ml saline, via oxygen-driven jet nebulizer

Steroids are commenced
> Hydrocortisone 200 mg intravenously or
> Prednisolone 30–60 mg orally

If **life-threatening features** are present:
> Immediately notify anaesthetist and medical on-call team
> Add ipratropium 0.5 mg to the nebulized beta agonist
> Consider **xanthine therapy**, if not already on xanthines
> **Aminophylline** 250 mg (6 mg/kg) over 20 minutes intravenously, followed by an infusion at 0.5 mg/kg/hour
> Obtain **portable chest X-ray** to look for pneumothorax
> Intubate and commence assisted ventilation if:

- Progressive exhaustion
- Progressive CO_2 retention
- Respiratory arrest

All patients with acute severe asthma require referral to the medical on-call team
Patients who do not fulfil the above criteria should be assessed individually, noting:
> Response of symptoms and peak flow to inhaled nebulized beta agonist

>

> Acute Asthma

Subsequent history taking should elicit warnings of decompensation and loss of control:

- Sleep disturbance
- Reduced exercise tolerance
- Increased need for bronchodilator use
- Decreasing effectiveness of bronchodilator treatment
- Fall in peak flow

All patients with milder asthma who show the above features should also be referred to the on-call medical team

Patients who are being sent home:

Should be observed at least 1 hour after completion of nebulizer therapy

Almost invariably require a short course of systemic steroid

Must be advised to see their GP at the earliest convenient moment for review of the clinical condition, or to return to the A&E department if symptoms recur

Pneumonia

Community acquired pneumonia can lead to A&E attendance with acute symptoms.

The history allows categorization into either of two broad categories:

TYPICAL PNEUMONIA

Sudden onset of:

- Cough
- Fever
- Chills
- Mucoid, purulent or blood-stained sputum
- Pleuritic chest pain
- Shortness of breath
- Wheeze
- Confusion (particularly in the elderly)

Localized chest signs

ATYPICAL PNEUMONIA

Gradual (subacute) onset, over 3–5 days, of:

- Malaise
- Fever
- Chills
- Headache
- Myalgia
- Arthralgia

These symptoms predominate over respiratory symptoms, which include:

Delayed onset of dry cough

Chest pain

Minimal or disproportionate chest signs

ASSESSMENT

In all cases, vital signs must be documented

Pulse oximetry is routinely required

Thorough chest auscultation is required

>

> Pneumonia

INVESTIGATIONS
Venous blood
FBC, U&E
Culture
Plasma serology (for atypical pneumonia)
Sputum
Gram stain
Culture
Chest X-ray
12-lead ECG, if irregular pulse noted

Markers of severe illness at presentation help in the decision to admit:

- Age over 60 years
- Confusion
- Respiratory rate over 30/minute
- Diastolic blood pressure less than 60 mmHg
- Atrial fibrillation of new onset
- Signs of involvement of more than one lobe
- White cell count
  $< 4 \times 10^9/l$
  or
  $> 20 \times 10^9/l$
- Blood urea > 7 mmol/l
- Multilobe involvement on chest X-ray

TYPICAL CHEST X-RAY FINDINGS
Consolidation
Opacity with ill-defined edge, unless marginated by pleura
Air bronchogram (branching linear transradiancies)
No volume change

MANAGEMENT
Antimicrobial therapy as either outpatient or on inpatient basis (if severe illness)

Spontaneous Pneumothorax

FEATURES

Sudden onset of severe unilateral pleuritic chest pain and shortness of breath often in a young adult

There may be a history of previous similar episodes

The findings on **EXAMINATION** include:

- Tachypnoea
- Asymmetrical chest expansion
- Diminished or absent breath sounds
- Hyper-resonant percussion note
- Tracheal shift
  and occasionally
- Subcutaneous emphysema
- Clicking noise on left side of chest synchronous with heart beat

ASSESSMENT includes:

- Vital signs
- Pulse oximetry
- Chest X-ray; ask for expiratory films which are better for visualizing small pneumothoraces

Drainage is indicated in the following situations:

- Tension pneumothorax
- If causing shortness of breath
- Moderate to large: occupies over one-third of transverse diameter of hemithorax at level of hilum
- Bilateral
- Associated haemothorax
- Increasing size in spite of conservative management
- Complicating chronic obstructive airways disease

Intercostal intubation is the traditional method of treatment. There may be a place for aspiration in certain situations.

>

> Spontaneous Pneumothorax

INTERCOSTAL TUBE

Site
  4th or 5th intercostal space just behind anterior axillary
   line preferred
  2nd intercostal space in midclavicular line

Size
  Infant 14–20 French
  Children 20–28 French
  Adolescent or adult 28–42 French
  A Heimlich flutter valve is useful for transportation of
   the patient

No treatment is needed if:

The pneumothorax is shallow (less than 20% collapse of
  lung)
  There are no symptoms

In these circumstances weekly follow-up with a chest X-ray
  is needed until the pleural air is completely absorbed

The **CHEST X-RAY FINDINGS** include:

A visceral pleural line
Air in the pleura, marked by a hyperlucent area devoid of
  lung markings
Lobar or lung collapse
Mediastinal and cardiac shift to the opposite side

Tension Pneumothorax

Tension pneumothorax is a lethal condition if untreated. Progressive air entrapment in the pleural space leads to loss of lung volume and compression of the great veins and heart, impairing venous return and cardiac filling.

The characteristic **FEATURES**, which may be associated with chest trauma, but may complicate any cause of spontaneous pneumothorax, include a combination of:

Progressive ventilatory failure
- Respiratory distress
- Cyanosis
- Failure of artificial ventilation
- High resistance to lung inflation
- Respiratory arrest

Progressive circulatory failure
- Tachycardia
- Hypotension
- Distended neck veins
- Cardiac arrest

Asymmetrical chest findings
- Hyper-resonance
- Absent breath sounds
- Progressive tracheal shift to the opposite side

Sign of air leak
- Palpable subcutaneous emphysema

Treatment is on clinical suspicion, prior to obtaining chest X-rays

Aspirate air from the 2nd intercostal space anteriorly in the midclavicular line, followed by intercostal intubation and post-intubation chest X-rays

Refer for admission

Haemoptysis

This is a relatively uncommon presentation as an isolated symptom in the A&E department unless the bleeding is massive.

The initial assessment should be aimed at determining the haemodynamic status of the patient, as determined by general observation and by recording of vital signs.

Clinical examination of the cardiovascular and respiratory systems should be carried out.

The initial investigations include:

Venous blood: FBC
Chest X-ray
Arterial blood gases

Initial management of the patient with massive haemoptysis consists of:

Venous access
Volume replacement
Lying on the side on which the lung is bleeding to avoid aspiration into the other lung. Head-down tilt
No sedation must be given

Medical referral is indicated with a view to early rigid bronchoscopy
If the bleeding is uncontrollable, endotracheal Intubation should be performed, preferably with a double-lumen endotracheal tube
Early endotracheal intubation is also required with an impaired gag reflex to prevent continued airway soiling
Further assessment of the cause of haemoptysis is facilitated by noting associated symptoms and signs:

● Pleuritic chest pain
Pneumonia
Pulmonary embolism
Chest trauma

>

> Haemoptysis

- Shortness of breath
    Pulmonary embolism
    Neoplasm
- Wheezing
    Bilateral: chronic obstructive airway disease
    Unilateral: neoplasm
                aspirated foreign body
- Pre-existing heart disease, especially mitral valve disease
- Presence of other sites of bleeding: coagulation disorders

MANAGEMENT

Minor episodes of haemoptysis can be treated or investigated on an outpatient basis in the absence of other reasons for admission

Massive haemoptysis requires inpatient management

Acute Exacerbation of Chronic Obstructive Airway Disease

This is a common cause for A&E attendance.

An acute exacerbation can be defined by an increase in the amount and purulence of sputum, associated with increased shortness of breath.

The usual **PRECIPITANTS** are:

- Respiratory infection
- Use of sedatives
- Cardiac failure
- Spontaneous pneumothorax
- Stoppage of maintenance medication

Initial **ASSESSMENT** is for:

- Vital signs
- Peak expiratory flow
- Colour
- Signs of respiratory distress

Initial **MANAGEMENT** includes:

Controlled oxygen therapy
24–28% oxygen by Venturi mask or nasal catheter at 2 litres/minute flow rate
Check ABGs after 30 minutes

Antimicrobial therapy
Amoxycillin

Nebulized bronchodilators if wheezing present

INVESTIGATIONS include:

Venous blood: FBC
Chest X-ray
Sputum: culture
12-lead ECG

Admission may be required for severe symptoms. Many patients are well compensated in spite of central cyanosis and grossly abnormal arterial blood gases. These patients should not be artificially ventilated as they become ventilator dependent.

Smoke Inhalation Injury

FEATURES

- Closed space flame burns
- Extrication from smoke-filled room, often unconscious
- Hoarse voice or loss of voice
- Singed nasal and eyebrow hairs
- Expectoration of soot
- Inspiratory stridor
- Intraoral heat injury
- Soot in nares and pharynx

ASSESSMENT

- Airway patency
- Breathing
- Venous blood: carboxyhaemoglobin on arrival
- Arterial blood gases
- Chest X-ray
- Commence 60% oxygen by face mask
- Check eyes for corneal abrasions (due to soot particles) with fluorescein staining
- Refer for admission

4 Neurological emergencies

The Unconscious Patient

The initial management consists of supporting vital functions while simultaneously attempting to determine the causes of unconsciousness.

The recommended sequence of events in A&E is as follows:

1. Ensure **airway patency**, simultaneously immobilizing the neck if trauma is likely

    Remove solid material and dentures from mouth

    Suction with rigid wide-bore sucker to remove blood, mucus and vomit from mouth

    Oral airway

2. Check **adequacy of ventilation**

    Auscultate over both lungs

    Pulse oximetry to look for tissue hypoxia

    Intubate and ventilate if spontaneous ventilation is inadequate

    Otherwise, give 60% oxygen by face mask

3. Document **vital signs**

    Heart rate

    Respiratory rate

    Blood pressure

    Temperature (use low reading thermometer if hypothermia is likely)

4. Establish **level of consciousness**, using **Glasgow Coma Scale**

5. Establish **venous access**

    At the same time take venous blood for:

    FBC

    U&E: glucose, alcohol (if relevant)

    Culture (if sepsis likely)

    Smear for malarial parasites (recent travel to malarial zone)

    Save specimen for toxic screen in heparinized bottle

6. Determine **bedside blood glucose** using BM Stix

    If low, give 50 ml 50% dextrose (25 g) intravenously, preceded by thiamine 100 mg intravenously if patient a known chronic alcoholic   >

> The Unconscious Patient

7. Consider the need for **specific antidotes**
   Naloxone: especially if pinpoint pupils
   Flumazenil: benzodiazepine overdose
8. Ensure a **history** is obtained before the ambulance personnel depart regarding the circumstances in which the patient was found. Obtain any relevant past medical history from accompanying friends or relatives.
9. If the patient is of unknown identity, check pockets for cards, medication, syringes and suicide notes. Look for Medic-Alert bracelets or necklaces.
10. Once the airway patency is ensured and breathing and circulation stabilized, a formal head-to-toe examination is performed, looking for:
    - Evidence of head injury
    - Odour on breath, e.g. alcohol, acetone
    - Pupil size and light reactions
    - Optic fundi: subhyaloid haemorrhage, papilloedema
    - Discharge or bleeding from ears (including otoscopy)
    - Abnormal movements or postures adopted by the limbs
    - Neck stiffness
    - Injection marks on the skin
    - Skin rash
    - Heart murmurs
    - Muscle tone in all four limbs
    - Deep tendon jerks
    - Plantar responses

DEFINITIVE MANAGEMENT

All patients will require admission
Further investigations while in A&E are guided by the category into which the patient can be assigned on the basis of initial assessment:

>

> The Unconscious Patient

Coma with meningeal signs

1. And focal neurological signs
CT/MRI scan
Usual causes:
- Intracerebral haematoma
- Subarachnoid haemorrhage with haematoma or infarction
- Chronic infection

2. No focal neurological signs
Lumbar puncture (LP)
or computed tomography (CT) followed by LP
Usual causes:
- Meningitis
- Encephalitis
- Subarachnoid haemorrhage

Coma without meningeal signs

1. And focal signs
CT scan
Mass lesion
Cerebral infarction

2. No focal signs
Metabolic or anoxic-ischaemic encephalopathy
Venous blood: U&E, glucose, alcohol
Toxic screen
Carboxyhaemoglobin
Arterial blood: ABGs

Stroke Assessment

The following questions must be answered:

IS IT A STROKE?

Sudden onset
Focal neurological deficit
Symptoms lasting more than 24 hours or resulting in death before 24 hours
Symptoms of non-traumatic vascular origin

WHAT IS THE UNDERLYING PATHOLOGICAL PROCESS?

1. Embolism

No warning
Sudden onset
Maximum deficit at onset
Clinically evident source of embolus, e.g. atrial fibrillation
Evidence of other organ involvement
Retention of consciousness
No headache
No neck stiffness

2. Haemorrhage

Warning headache
Sudden onset
Severe headache
Rapid loss of consciousness in some cases
Neck stiffness
Severe neurological deficit
Hypertension

3. Thrombosis

Warning transient ischaemic attack(s)
Gradual onset
Stepwise progression
Mild headache sometimes
No neck stiffness
Retention of consciousness
Coexisting evidence of peripheral vascular disease

>

> Stroke Assessment

WHAT IS THE ARTERIAL AREA AFFECTED?
Carotid
Vertebro-basilar

NON-VASCULAR LESIONS CAN MIMIC STROKE and must be considered in the differential diagnosis.

Mass lesions
   Subdural haematoma
   Primary intracranial tumours
   Metastases
   Cerebral abscess
Metabolic disturbances
   Hypoglycaemia
   Hyperosmolar states
   Hypernatremia/hyponatremia
Infections
   Meningitis
   Neurosyphilis
Post-ictal paralysis
Hysteria
Migraine

Investigations in the stroke patient

Full blood count
   Polycythaemia
   Thrombocytopenia
   Thrombocytosis
ESR
   Vasculitis
   Bacterial endocarditis
Blood glucose
   Hypoglycaemia
   Hyperglycaemia
Urea and electrolytes
Syphilis serology
12-lead ECG

>

Chest X-ray
  Bronchogenic carcinoma
  Cardiac source of embolus

Features suggestive of non-vascular lesion:

Mimicking stroke

- Age under 45 years
- Absence of risk factors for stroke
- Prolonged and/or discontinuous evolution of neurological deficit
- Associated seizures
- Fluctuating conscious level
- Pyrexia at presentation
- Papilloedema

Indications for CT scan in stroke patient:

- Doubtful diagnosis (stroke mimics)
- Cerebellar stroke suspected
- Differentiation between primary intracerebral haemorrhage and cerebral infarction where anticoagulation or thrombolytic therapy is under consideration

MANAGEMENT

All patients require medical referral

Transient Ischaemic Attacks (TIA)

CAROTID TIA

Ipsilateral monocular blindness (amaurosis fugax)
Contralateral hemiparesis
Contralateral hemianaesthesia
Aphasia (if dominant cerebral hemisphere involved)

VERTEBRO-BASILAR TIA

Diplopia
Vertigo
Ataxia
Bilateral motor and/or sensory deficit
Nausea and vomiting
Deafness and tinnitus
Dysarthria
Dysphagia
Cortical blindness

Features required for **DIAGNOSIS** of TIA:

- Sudden onset
- Focal neurological dysfunction
- Complete recovery
- Lasts less than 24 hours

Non-focal symptoms which are not features of a TIA:

- Isolated loss of consciousness (syncope)
- Faintness (presyncope)
- Dizziness
- Confusion
- Incontinence
- Visual blurring

ASSESSMENT of a patient with TIA should include examination of:

Optic fundi

Retinal arteriolar microemboli

Vascular system

Pulse and blood pressure in both arms

>

> Transient Ischaemic Attacks (TIA)

Auscultation for
  Carotid and subclavian bruits
  Cardiac murmurs

INVESTIGATIONS

Venous blood
  FBC, erythrocyte sedimentation rate (ESR)
  Sickle test
  U&E, glucose
  Syphilis serology
Chest X-ray
12-lead ECG
Specialized
  Ultrasound of carotid
  Echocardiography

MANAGEMENT

All TIAs should be referred for medical follow-up and
  investigation
Blind treatment with low-dose aspirin may lead to the
  neglect of potentially treatable causes

Isolated Seizures

Patients who exhibit seizure activity in public places are almost invariably brought to the nearest A&E department. This might be inappropriate if the patient is known to be epileptic and the seizure is self-limiting. However, it is unlikely that this situation will alter in the near future.

Confronted with an individual who has allegedly recently had a fit, the initial assessment should ensure airway patency, adequacy of breathing and stable vital signs. The single most important tool in the diagnosis of an unwitnessed seizure is a good history from a reliable eye witness.

The questions that need to be asked are:

- Was the attack epileptic?
- If so, what type was it?
- What is the likely cause?

HISTORY

The following points should be elucidated:

Is the patient known to be an epileptic?

If so, what treatment has been prescribed?

What is the usual frequency of fits?

Is compliance likely to be adequate?

Was the present episode similar to ones occurring in the past?

If the patient is not known to be epileptic, a detailed history is vital stressing the following points:

Were any warning symptoms perceived by the patient?

Were there any likely precipitating factors?

What was the patient doing at the onset?

What were the features witnessed?

Was there loss of consciousness?

Did the limbs twitch? If so, was this generalized or localized to one or more limbs, or initially localized before becoming generalized?

How long did the attack last?

What was the patient like afterwards?

>

> Isolated Seizures

Post-ictal drowsiness, confusion and headache signify a grand mal seizure

Features associated with a grand mal seizure include:

The attack often occurs when the patient is alone or asleep. Indeed, the patient may be first discovered in a drowsy or confused state after the seizure has subsided

There is usually no precipitant

A warning aura may be present

The patient may bite his or her tongue

Incontinence for urine and/or faeces may occur

The patient may sustain injury, e.g. facial or scalp bruising, dislocated shoulder, spinal trauma, etc.

Tonic or tonic–clonic movements involve all four extremities

Breathing may be stertorous

Central cyanosis may develop

On cessation the patient is drowsy and confused

A good history is diagnostic of a grand mal seizure. Every attempt must be made to get as much information as possible at this stage, as subsequent recall may be less efficient.

Once a seizure is confirmed, further **HISTORY** taking must be directed to ascertaining whether an intracranial lesion is likely. This would help decide the need for urgent investigations.

A history of headache, vomiting and visual disturbance may suggest raised intracranial pressure

A history of a coexisting or previous malignancy might suggest the possibility of intracranial metastases

A history of recent cranial trauma is also significant

Documentation of alcohol intake is important as alcohol may be related to seizure disorder in a number of ways

>

> Isolated Seizures

Features suggesting a possible structural aetiology include:
- Adult-onset seizure
- Aura at onset
- Associated recent onset neurological symptoms
    Headache
    Nausea and vomiting
    Dysphasia
    Limb weakness or numbness
- Focal onset seizures
- Post-ictal focal features such as hemiparesis, dysphasia or unilateral hypoesthesia

Specific features to be noted on examination include:
- Alertness
- Glasgow Coma Score
- Airway patency
- Breathing
- Circulatory status including vital signs
- Pupillary reactions
- Signs of raised intracranial pressure
- Papilloedema
- Signs of meningeal irritation
- Focal neurological deficits
    Hemiparesis
    Hemianaesthesia
    Visual field defects
- Signs of injury, especially orofacial, scalp, spine, limbs

MANAGEMENT

All patients with adult-onset isolated seizures not related to a specific precipitant, e.g. hypoglycaemia or alcohol withdrawal, need specialist referral.

An isolated seizure does not lead to a diagnosis of epilepsy and does not warrant drug treatment.

Following isolated seizures all patients should not drive and should notify the DVLA. This advice should be recorded in the clinical notes. Patients should also be >

> Isolated Seizures

advised about dangerous occupations (e.g. working at heights on scaffolding) and unsuitable recreation (e.g. swimming unaccompanied).

Attendants/relatives should be advised how to deal with a further seizure should one occur.

INVESTIGATIONS

The role of investigations in seizure disorder are limited and are directed towards detecting the cause.

Recommended initial investigations include:

- Metabolic
    Urea and electrolytes
    Blood glucose
    Serum calcium
- Radiological
    Chest X-ray: if bronchogenic carcinoma suspected
    Skull X-ray is of limited value
        If an intracranial space-occupying lesion is suspected, CT or magnetic resonance imaging (MRI) scanning is indicated
- 12-lead ECG

Status Epilepticus

Status epilepticus is defined as a seizure lasting over 30 minutes or several distinct episodes without consciousness being regained.

MANAGEMENT

The priority in management is rapid termination of seizure activity, while protecting vital functions

IMMEDIATE CARE

The airway must be cleared of blood and secretions by a rigid sucker.

The patient must be positioned in the lateral decubitus position to prevent occlusion of the airway by the tongue

Intravenous access must be secured

Pulse oximetric monitoring must be commenced

Do not attempt to restrain

DEFINITIVE CARE

Anticonvulsant therapy

First line:

Diazepam 10 mg over 2 minutes (0.25 mg/kg in a child) intravenously (IV)

or

Clonazepam 1 mg over 2 minutes IV

Second line:

Paraldehyde 10 ml intramuscularly (IM) (5 ml into each buttock)

or

Chlormethiazole (0.8% solution) as IV infusion; 50–100 ml in 10 minutes followed by up to 100 ml/hour

or

Phenytoin 50 mg/minute IV with ECG monitoring up to a total of 1000 mg (15–18 mg/kg in normal saline)

Third line:

Notify anaesthetist and ITU.

Thiopentone IV, muscle relaxants and assisted ventilation

>

> Status Epilepticus

INVESTIGATIONS

Venous blood
Glucose, U&E
Calcium
Anticonvulsant levels (where appropriate)

Arterial blood
ABGs

Headache

Headache is a common symptom in the community and often self-treated. However, acute severe headache and more rarely episodic or subacute progressive headache may constitute reasons for attendance at an A&E department. It follows that the likelihood of detecting significant underlying pathology is higher in patients with headache attending an A&E department.

For practical purposes the following **clinical patterns of headache** may be recognized:

1. **Acute severe headache**
   Meningitis
   Subarachnoid haemorrhage
   Extracranial causes
      Acute angle closure glaucoma
      Paranasal sinusitis
2. **Recurrent episodic headache**
   Migraine
   Cluster headache
   Headache associated with paroxysmal hypertension
      e.g. phaeochromocytoma
3. **Progressive subacute headache** (sinister pattern of headache)
   Intracranial space-occupying lesion
4. **Chronic continuous headache**
   Tension headache

ASSESSMENT of the patient with headache comprises the following essential steps:

1. **History**
   Duration of symptoms
      In general, the longer the duration the less the likelihood of serious pathology
   Previous episodes of similar symptoms
   Relationship of onset to physical exertion or coitus
   Progression of symptoms
   Radiation to the neck and/or back

>

> **Headache**

Fever
Associated symptoms
Vomiting
Visual symptoms
Ataxia
Diurnal variation in severity of symptoms
Family history of subarachnoid haemorrhage
Early morning headache is particularly suggestive of
raised intracranial pressure

2. **Physical examination**
Mental state
Alertness and orientation
Speech
Blood pressure
Temperature
Temporal arterial pulsations and tenderness
Skull bruits
Signs of meningeal irritation
Neck stiffness
Kernig's sign
Gait and stance
Visual fields and acuity
Optic fundi
Paranasal sinus tenderness
Ear drums
Dentition

INDICATIONS FOR CT SCANNING in the presence of
headache:

- Signs of meningeal irritation
- Depressed level of consciousness
- Lateralizing or localizing neurological signs
- Papilloedema

Subarachnoid Haemorrhage

Commonly **PRESENTS** with:

Acute severe headache, associated with vomiting, pain in the neck or back, photophobia

There may be a history of recent similar minor episodes (herald bleeds)

Occasionally the presentation is with rapid loss of consciousness

INITIAL ASSESSMENT comprises:

Assessing airway patency, adequacy of breathing and circulatory status if unconscious

Vital signs

Glasgow Coma Score

SPECIFIC FINDINGS to be looked for include:

Signs of meningeal irritation

Subhyaloid haemorrhages on examination of the optic fundi

Intracranial bruits on auscultation of the skull

A neurological examination to look for focal deficits

FOCAL SIGNS that may be present include:

3rd cranial nerve palsy

Aneurysms at junction of posterior communicating and internal carotid arteries

Hemiplegia with or without aphasia

Aneurysms at first major bifurcation of the middle cerebral artery

Monocular blindness

INVESTIGATIONS

Venous blood: FBC, U&E

12-lead ECG: often abnormalities due to myocardial ischaemia or cardiac arrhythmias coexist

CT scan

This shows subarachnoid blood in 90% scanned within 24 hours of onset of symptoms

>

> Subarachnoid Haemorrhage

Scan may also reveal intracerebral, subdural or intraventricular haematoma

With contrast enhancement, the responsible aneurysm or arteriovenous malformation may be visible

If the CT scan is normal, lumbar puncture must be performed in the absence of any contraindications. This will reveal blood-stained cerebrospinal fluid with xanthochromic supernatant

Neurosurgical referral and subsequent four-vessel angiography are needed if the diagnosis is confirmed

TREATMENT that might be needed while in A&E includes:

For **headache**
Codeine phosphate 60 mg stat and 4–6 hourly orally or intramuscularly

For **vomiting**
Metoclopramide 10 mg intramuscularly

For **seizures**
Diazepam intravenously

CONTRAINDICATIONS TO LUMBAR PUNCTURE

Papilloedema
Focal neurological deficit

Meningitis

Meningitis is a serious, potentially fatal illness that often presents with non-specific symptoms. Presentation varies with age and immune status of the patient. A high index of clinical suspicion is required to ensure the diagnosis is not missed.

The **FEATURES AT PRESENTATION** include:

Adults

Typical presentation

Acute onset of:

- Fever
- Headache
- Drowsiness
- Vomiting
- Photophobia
- Neck or back pain
- Neck stiffness

Atypical presentation

Irritability or behaviour change may occur in the young, the elderly and the immunosuppressed

Infants and children

- Refusal to feed
- Vomiting
- Drowsiness
- Irritability
- Altered high-pitched cry
- Raised anterior fontanelle tension
- Fever
- Convulsions
- Stiff neck: detected by asking child to kiss knees

A pleomorphic petechial rash commencing on the trunk and spreading centrifugally strongly suggests meningococcal infection. The lesions may enlarge, coalesce, ulcerate and be complicated by necrosis. Rapid evolution of the rash often occurs. In these circumstances **benzylpenicillin** must be administered immediately >

> Meningitis

(1200 mg for adults and children aged over 10 years; 600 mg for children aged 1–9 years; and 300 mg for children aged under 1 year).

MANAGEMENT

Once meningitis is suspected, the patient should be referred to the on-call medical or paediatric team as appropriate. Initial investigations include:

Venous blood
    FBC
    U&E
    Culture
Lumbar puncture
    CSF: Gram stain
           Glucose
           Protein
           Culture

Acute Ataxia

The acute onset of unsteadiness may be alarming, especially to people accompanying the patient, leading to A&E attendance.

The abuse of alcohol is a common reversible cause of ataxia in the A&E department.

The presence of associated symptoms helps categorization according to cause:

With **drowsiness**, but no features of raised intracranial pressure:
Toxic encephalopathy, caused by
Alcohol
Phenytoin toxicity
Sedative hypnotics, e.g. benzodiazepines

With signs of **meningeal irritation** or **raised intracranial pressure**:
Posterior cranial fossa neoplasms, haemorrhage or abscess (usually cerebellar)
Lead encephalopathy
Bacterial meningitis
Viral meningoencephalitis

With **vomiting, nausea and headache, but no evidence of raised intracranial pressure**:
Migraine
Labyrinth
Labyrinthitis

With **weakness**:
Guillain Barré syndrome
Acute transverse myelitis

Limb Weakness

Determination of the cause of limb weakness is based on elucidation of:

Mode of onset: whether acute or acute on chronic
Distribution: whether involving one limb
one upper and lower limb
all four limbs
Whether upper motor neurone weakness (spasticity, hyper-reflexia, (extensor plantar responses)
lower motor neurone weakness (flaccidity, fasciculations, hyporeflexia; wasting is a late feature)
muscular (wasting, hypotonia, reduced or absent reflexes)
Whether cranial nerve palsies coexist
The precise distribution of the motor deficit
Whether isolated muscle
muscle group
myotome
entire limb (if so, in which muscle groups is the loss predominant, e.g. flexor or extensor)

Some **COMMON PATTERNS OF LIMB WEAKNESS** can be identified as a result:

Unilateral upper motor neurone lesions
Cerebral and brainstem lesions
Cervical cord hemisection

Weakness of both lower limbs
Upper motor neurone: spinal cord lesions
Lower motor neurone: cauda equina lesions

Single limb weakness
Lower motor neurone: peripheral neuropathy, radiculopathy

Usually medical referral is required
Motor deficits secondary to trauma require orthopaedic follow-up

Acute Dystonic Reactions

Often cause bizarre presentations

A high index of clinical suspicion is necessary as the patient may not connect the symptoms to current medication

FEATURES

- Neck pain and stiffness
- Spasmodic torticollis
- Painful trismus
- Tongue protrusion
- Neck retraction
- Inability to speak
- Opisthotonus
- Choking
- Oculogyric crisis

The **MEDICATIONS RESPONSIBLE** include:

- Phenothiazines
- Butyrophenones
- Metoclopramide
- Antihistamines
- Domperidone

Usually the clinical context is of treatment for psychosis or anti-emetic therapy

TREATMENT

- Benztropine 1–2 mg intravenously
- Procyclidine 10 mg intravenously

5 Psychiatric emergencies

Mental State Assessment

This is crucial to the adequate assessment of mentally ill patients. With a little practice, valuable information can be rapidly elicited. This leads to better liaison with psychiatric services, especially when internal communication is via the phone.

APPEARANCE

General appearance
State of dress
Grooming
Make-up
Cleanliness

Facial expression
Sadness
Anger
Distress

SPEECH

Amount
Flow
Content

MOOD

Depression
Anxiety

THOUGHT PROCESSES

Structure
Circumstantiality
Loose associations
Flight of ideas

Content
Delusions
Phobias
Ideas of reference
Obsessions

>

COGNITIVE FUNCTION

Level of consciousness
Orientation in time, place and person
Memory
Abstract thinking
Calculation

PERCEPTUAL FUNCTION

Illusions
Hallucinations

INSIGHT AND JUDGEMENT

Mental Health Act 1983

Has 149 sections

Sections relevant to A&E practice are:

1. Related to admission for **assessment**

   Section 2　　　Application for admission for assessment or assessment and treatment

   28 days

   Section 4　　　Emergency Order for Assessment

   72 hours

   Section 136　　Mentally disordered person found in a public place and brought to the department by the police

2. **Treatment orders**

   Section 3　　　Compulsory Admission for Treatment

   6 months

Sections 2 and 3 require the signatures of two doctors (one approved) and the nearest relative or a social worker

Section 4 requires the signature of one doctor and one relative or social worker

Deliberate Self-Harm

Asessment of suicidal intent is a vital part of the overall management of all patients presenting after deliberate self-harm. This may have to be deferred if there are any life-threatening physical complications requiring urgent treatment.

The capability to assess suicidal intent should be within the province of all doctors working in A&E departments. All threats of suicide by a patient should be taken seriously.

CIRCUMSTANTIAL INDICATORS OF SERIOUS SUICIDE ATTEMPT

- Active preparation, e.g. hoarding drugs
- Final acts in anticipation of death
    Making a will
    Settling financial affairs
- Planning to be alone
- Timing attempt to avoid intervention by others
- Taking precautions against discovery, e.g. locking door
- Writing a suicide note
- Not seeking help after the attempt
- Selection of violent or medically serious method with high lethality, e.g. hanging, shooting, jumping from a height

ASSESSMENT OF SURVIVOR OF ATTEMPTED SUICIDE

- Nature of attempt
    Method used: self poisoning, hanging, drowning, shooting, car exhaust fume exposure
    Circumstances of attempt
- Reasons for attempt
    Problems
    Motives, including suicidal intent
- Psychiatric disorder
    Depressive symptoms (loss of sleep, appetite, interest in sex)

>

> **Deliberate Self-Harm**

    Symptoms of psychosis
- Alcohol abuse

RISK FACTORS FOR COMPLETED SUICIDE AFTER ATTEMPTED SUICIDE
Socio-demographic
Older age group

Male sex

Unemployed

Single, separated or divorced

Living alone

No friends

Certain occupations, e.g. doctor
Circumstances of attempt
Clinical factors
Psychiatric disorders

    Depression

    Schizophrenia

Chronic physical illness causing severe disability or severe pain

Alcohol/substance abuse

Personality disorder

CHARACTERISTICS OF PARASUICIDE

- Female
- Social class V
- Alcohol abuse
- Personality disorder (sociopathic, histrionic, passive dependent)
- Younger age group
- Unemployed
- Criminal record
- Drug addiction
- Previous parasuicide

MANAGEMENT

All patients with suicidal intent should be referred to a psychiatrist for assessment and management.

Violence

Violence is an increasing problem in A&E departments, especially in inner cities. Training to recognize the potentially violent individual, to avert violence, and to deal adequately with the violent incident are mandatory for all A&E personnel, both medical and nursing. Many hospitals now provide in-house training and have policy documents for dealing with threatened or actual violence.

The usual **CAUSES** of violent behaviour include:

Drug intoxication
   Alcohol
   Amphetamines
   Phencyclidine
Drug withdrawal
   Heroin
   Alcohol
   Barbiturates
Psychosis
   Schizophrenia
   Mania
   Dementia
Metabolic encephalopathy
   Hypoglycaemia
   Uraemia
Seizure disorder
   Post-ictal confusion
   Temporal lobe epilepsy
Sociopathic personality disorder

When dealing with a violent or potentially violent patient, ensure you are accompanied and have access to exits and alarm systems such as panic buttons.

PREDICTORS OF VIOLENT BEHAVIOUR

- Previous history of violence
- Alcohol and drug abuse
- Paranoid thinking

>

> Violence

- Behavioural clues
  - Non-verbal
    - Physical closeness or contact
    - Gestures
    - Facial expressions
  - Verbal
    - Threats of violence

MANAGEMENT

Initially attempt **verbal restraint**, consisting of:

  Active listening, showing empathy and concern
  Keeping space between yourself and the patient
  Avoid intense eye contact
  Use a non-judgemental approach

If there is a risk of injury to a person or damage to property, **physical restraint** may be needed, often with the assistance of hospital security staff or the police.

Rarely, **chemical restraint** may be needed, such as haloperidol 5–10 mg intramuscularly.

Acute Schizophrenia

The acutely psychotic patient is often brought to the A&E department by a concerned friend, relative or member of the public.

The usual **FEATURES** are:

Appearance and behaviour
   Bizarre dress
   Self-neglect
   Self-talking
   Inappropriate laughter

Speech
   Neologisms

Mood
   Normal or incongruous

Thought content
   Paranoid delusions, frequently persecutory
   Passivity experiences
   Thought broadcasting
   Thought insertion
   Thought withdrawal

Perceptual abnormalities
   Audible thoughts

Catatonic phenomena

Loss of insight

MANAGEMENT

Psychiatric referral is needed

Emergency parenteral medication may be needed to restrain a violent psychotic patient where verbal and physical restraint have failed. Thereafter, close monitoring of level of consciousness and of vital signs is required.

The usual preferred agent may be either:
   Chlorpromazine 25–50 mg intramuscularly
   Haloperidol 2–10 mg intramuscularly, repeated hourly
   Droperidol 5–20 mg intramuscularly

Procyclidine 5–10 mg intramuscularly may be given to prevent dystonic reactions

Factitious Disease

Factitious disease is characterized by the conscious production of signs or symptoms by the patient, with no gain, either economic or social, as a result of the simulation.

Factitious illness can cause considerable diagnostic difficulty in an A&E department.

The major categories of factitious illness include:

- Simulated disease, e.g. myocardial infarction, renal colic
- Self-induced disease, e.g. insulin-induced hypoglycaemia
- Aggravation of pre-existing disease, e.g. labile or brittle diabetes, pseudoseizures complicating genuine epilepsy
- Munchausen's syndrome

  This condition not infrequently confronts the junior A&E doctor, especially out of hours

  The typical features are:

  An unaccompanied male of low socio-economic class

  A dramatic presentation of acute illness, e.g. acute abdomen, chest pain, ureteric colic

  A history of multiple hospitalizations and investigations and invasive procedures

  Disruptive behaviour

Factitious disease must be suspected with any dramatic or unusual illness in which the clinical features are variable or inconsistent and where the patient appears particularly knowledgeable and demands specific treatment, e.g. narcotic analgesia.

If a definitive diagnosis can be made, no further physical interventions should be carried out. The patient should be told that the deception has been discovered and offered psychiatric help, upon which self-discharge typically takes place.

Bereavement

Death is not an infrequent event in an A&E department.

Staff dealing with the recently bereaved must be trained in breaking bad news.

PREPARATION

Introduce yourself
Determine relationship of person(s) to whom you are speaking and the deceased

ENVIRONMENT

Have a nurse present
Ensure privacy
Sit down
Make tissues available

GIVING INFORMATION

Ensure that the death of the patient is announced in unambiguous terms at the outset
Use frequent eye contact
Allow for spontaneous expressions of anguish, fear or anger

CONTINUING CARE

Inform GP of patient's death
Offer counselling where available
Provide information regarding need for notifying Coroner
Be aware of possible organ donation by patients carrying donor cards

Panic Attack

This is an acute episode of anxiety of sudden onset and often dramatic presentation.

A variety of somatic complaints may occur:

- Palpitations
- Chest pain
- Paraesthesiae in the limbs (often progressing to tetany)
- Hyperventilation
- Headache
- Tremor of the limbs
- Fatigue
- Sweating
- Dryness of the mouth
- Frequency of passing urine

The age of the patient is almost invariably under 35 years

MANAGEMENT

Reassure the patient

Encourage rebreathing into a paper bag

Sedation may be needed, usually with administration of a benzodiazepine, such as diazepam, 5–10 mg orally

6 Toxicological emergencies

Acute Poisoning

GENERAL PRINCIPLES

Resuscitation and assessment should proceed simultaneously

The history is often not immediately available, and unreliable as to the amount and nature of substance(s) ingested and the time of ingestion

The immediate **PRIORITIES** are to:

Ensure airway patency

Intubation with a cuffed endotracheal tube is indicated if the gag reflex is abolished

Ensure adequate ventilation

Check circulatory status

Blood pressure, pulse rate

Obtain venous access

Plasma expanders if hypotensive

12-lead ECG followed by continuous ECG monitoring if arrhythmia present

Administer oxygen if hypoxic

Administer naloxone if respiratory depression and pinpoint pupils coexist

Consider the use of flumazenil for benzodiazepine overdose

Initial **INVESTIGATIONS** that may be needed include:

Venous blood

U&E

Paracetamol and salicylate levels

At least 4 hours post-ingestion

Always checked if patient unconscious

Save serum for toxic screen in heparinized bottle

Arterial blood: ABGs

12-lead ECG

When dealing with unfamiliar drugs or circumstances, the Regional Poisons Unit should be contacted for advice. In some A&E departments, direct access to a computerized database may be available. >

> Acute Poisoning

Initial **DECISIONS** involve the following steps:

1. Should the stomach be emptied?
    Toxic amount ingested under 1 hour ago
    Toxic amount of salicylate or tricyclic antidepressant
        ingested under 6 hours ago
    Not for caustic or hydrocarbon ingestion
2. If so, what method should be used?
    Gastric lavage
    Induced emesis (syrup of ipecacuanha)
3. Should further absorption be prevented?
    Oral activated charcoal
    Toxic ingestion under 1 hour ago
4. Should active elimination techniques be employed?
    Forced acid/alkaline diuresis
    Dialysis: haemodialysis/peritoneal dialysis
    Plasmapheresis
    Haemofiltration
    Exchange transfusion
5. Are specific antidotes required?
    Paracetamol: N-acetylcysteine
                        methionine
    Opiates: naloxone
    Heavy metals: chelating agents
    Carbon monoxide: oxygen
    Cholinesterase inhibitors: pralidoxime
        (Organophosphates): atropine
    Digoxin: digoxin-specific antibodies
    Warfarin: vitamin K
    Beta blockers: beta adrenergic agents
    Methanol: ethanol

Subsequent assessment should aim to determine the
underlying cause for the overdose, i.e. whether
    Accidental
    Deliberate self-harm
    Homicidal
    Child abuse

>

> Acute Poisoning

PHYSICAL SIGNS that may help determine the nature of the toxic agent(s) include:

- Smell on breath
- Pupil size and light reaction
- Skin bullae, venipuncture marks, bruising
- Dystonic reactions
- Oral burns
- Cardiac arrhythmias

Indications for **admission to hospital**:

- Intensive monitoring and supportive treatment needed
- Altered level of consciousness
- Specific antidotes required
- Suicidal intent
- Adolescent

Non-Toxic Ingestants

A variety of household objects and chemicals are non-toxic. Early identification of non-toxic ingestants may permit reassurance and early discharge from the A&E department, often by the triage nurse or nurse practitioner. These substances can be classified under the following headings:

DRUGS

Oral contraceptives
Vitamin supplements (without iron)
Antacids
Homeopathic preparations

HOUSEHOLD PRODUCTS

Soaps and detergents

Bubble bath
Fabric soakers, washing powder and flakes
Shaving foam and soaps
Scouring powders
Shampoo

Paints and markers

Chalk
Crayon
Felt-tip pens
Indelible markers
Inks
Pencils (graphite, colouring)
Watercolour paints for children

Cosmetics

Bath oils
Cream for hands, body and hair
Deodorants
Hair conditioner
Lipstick
Makeup for face and eyes
Suntan creams and lotions
Toothpaste
Talc

>

> Non-Toxic Ingestants

Bland skin creams
Zinc oxide
Calamine lotion
Petroleum jelly
Lanolin
Vaseline

Other
Candles
Modelling clay
Sweetening agents, e.g. saccharine
Thermometer contents (mercury, alcohol, glass)
Water-based pastes, gums and adhesives

Drug Abuse

Drug abusers may present to an A&E department for various reasons:

Primary care: many are unregistered with GPs or are transient, of no fixed abode

Secondary care for medical or psychiatric complications of drug abuse

Obtaining drugs by false pretext, for self-use or for sale to other addicts

When confronted with a known drug abuser, the following questions need to be asked:

Why has this patient come here?

What does he/she expect?

Drugs of potential abuse must never be prescribed for non-medical reasons

Does he/she have a medical problem for which investigation, treatment or admission is necessary?

Specific **ASSESSMENT** of the drug abuser includes:

- Type(s) of drug(s) used
- Method(s) of administration
- HIV/hepatitis B status if known
- Injection sites for evidence of infection or thrombosis
- Any ongoing or previous treatment for addiction
- Is pregnancy possible, if woman of child-bearing age?

Specific **MEDICAL COMPLICATIONS OF DRUG ABUSE** which lead to A&E attendance are:

Drug related

Overdose

Toxic psychosis

Withdrawal seizures

Injection related

Abscess(es), cellulitis

Thrombophlebitis

Acute arterial ischaemia with gangrene

Osteomyelitis

Septic arthritis

>

> **Drug Abuse**

Septicaemia
Allergic reactions
Pneumonia
Lung abscess
Viral hepatitis

When dealing with a drug addict:

Use a non-judgemental approach

Do not prescribe medication that is being demanded, for which there is no medical indication

Potentially violent patients may have to be removed physically by hospital security personnel or by the police

Take precautions against skin and ocular contamination If performing minor surgical procedures (use double gloves, eyeshield, gown or plastic overall)

Label all specimens as high risk

Notify the Home Office where appropriate using the forms provided

Be aware of local advice and treatment services for addicts

CONTROLLED DRUGS

Cocaine
Dextromoramide
Diamorphine (heroin)
Dipipanone
Hydrocodone
Hydromorphone
Levorphanol
Methadone
Morphine
Opium
Oxycodone
Pethidine
Phenazocine
Piritramide
Temazepam

>

INDICATIONS FOR PRESCRIBING CONTROLLED DRUGS TO A DRUG ABUSER

Relief of severe physical pain from an identifiable cause
Emergency treatment of withdrawal symptoms, particularly in pregnant females

Alcohol-Related Attendances in A&E

The effects of acute alcohol intoxication are particularly evident in A&E departments on Friday and Saturday nights. Alcohol-related attendances complicating chronic alcohol abuse can, however, occur at any time of day.

Wherever possible, an accurate history of the amount and frequency of alcohol consumption should be documented.

A history of alcohol consumption is ideally recorded in terms of units. 1 standard unit of alcohol is equivalent to:
    8 g absolute alcohol
    1 standard UK measure of spirits
    1 glass of sherry
    ½ pint of average strength beer
    1 glass of table wine

ACUTE PRESENTATIONS of alcohol abuse include:

Acute intoxication
Withdrawal syndromes
    Early mild (within 6-12 hours of abstinence)
    Acute alcoholic tremulousness (early morning shakes)
    Later major features (after 24–72 hours of abstinence)
Acute auditory hallucinosis
Grand mal seizures
Delirium tremens

The clinical features of alcohol intoxication are unreliable in determining the severity of ingestion. Most of the features are non-specific. They include:

- Smell of alcohol on the breath
- Slurred speech
- Euphoria
- Facial flushing with conjunctival redness
- Ataxic gait
- Increased activity
- Emotional lability
- Amnesia
- Coma, with severe intoxication

>

> Alcohol-Related Attendances in A&E

The **MANAGEMENT** of the acutely intoxicated is essentially supportive, with attention being given to airway status, adequacy of breathing and circulatory status. A careful search for injuries must be made. Coma must not be ascribed to alcohol if there are reasons to implicate trauma to the head or abdominal viscera. Alcoholics 'sleeping it off' in A&E must be periodically assessed, checking vital signs and neurological status, until they are awake. At the onset, plasma glucose must be checked as hypoglycaemia can frequently complicate acute intoxication.

The particular problems associated with alcohol intoxication that need to be considered in the A&E department include:

- Associated head, chest, neck, abdominal and limb injury
- Concurrent overdose of other drugs
- Association with road and workplace accidents
- Potential for violence
- Suicidal intent
- An association with seizures, which may be due to:
  Head injury, especially subdural haematoma
  Metabolic complications, e.g. hypoglycaemia
                                hyponatraemia
                                hypomagnesaemia

  Ethanol withdrawal
  Alcoholic brain disease

DELIRIUM TREMENS

This is a life-threatening withdrawal state that typically develops 3 to 5 days after ethanol withdrawal. The clinical features include:

- Acute confusional state
  Loss of orientation in time and place
  Clouding of consciousness
- Increased motor activity
  Tremulousness
  Purposeless activity
  Ataxia of gait

>

> Alcohol-Related Attendances in A&E

- Hallucinations, particularly visual
- Sympathetic hyperactivity
    - Sweating
    - Tachycardia
    - Mydriasis
    - Fever
    - Hypertension

MANAGEMENT

Check status of hydration and look for signs of infection

INVESTIGATIONS

Venous blood: FBC, U&E, glucose, liver function tests (LFTs)
Arterial blood: ABGs

SUPPORTIVE CARE

Commence intravenous infusion
Administer Parentrovite (water-soluble B and C vitamins)

SEDATION

Commence chlormethiazole infusion
Refer to on-call medical team for admission

Paracetamol Overdose

A common problem in A&E departments, often associated with parasuicide, paracetamol overdose is the most common cause of acute liver failure in the UK.

TREATMENT IS INDICATED FOR:

All patients with plasma paracetamol levels above the standard treatment line joining 200 mg/l at 4 hours post-ingestion and 50 mg/l at 12 hours post-ingestion on a nomogram

All patients ingesting a hepatotoxic dose
   i.e. over 5 g in a person aged 12 years or older
       over 150 mg/kg in a child

High-risk patients at half of the standard treatment line level

1. Glutathione deficiency
   Chronic alcoholism
   Anorexia nervosa
   HIV positive
2. On hepatic enzyme-inducing drugs
   e.g. anticonvulsants

Treatment depends on duration after ingestion of overdose

Less than 4 hours post-ingestion
Empty stomach by gastric lavage in an adult or induced emesis in a child
Blood at 4 hours for plasma paracetamol

4-8 hours post-ingestion
Take blood for plasma paracetamol levels
Antidote therapy for toxic levels

8–15 hours post-ingestion
Take venous blood for plasma paracetamol levels
Commence antidote immediately
Stop antidote if level below treatment line

Pregnant women are treated in the same way as other patients   >

> Paracetamol Overdose

Over 15 hours post-ingestion
Supportive treatment only
Check PTT and liver function daily until 4th day after ingestion

Note: Plasma levels are not useful in the presence of stuttering overdose (at several separate times).

ANTIDOTE THERAPY

N-acetylcysteine dose	Solvent volume (5% dextrose)	Infusion period
150 mg/kg	200 ml then	15 minutes
50 mg/kg	500 ml then	4 hours
50 mg/kg	500 ml then	8 hours
50 mg/kg	500 ml	8 hours

INDICATIONS FOR REFERRAL TO A LIVER UNIT

Prothrombin time in seconds greater than hours since overdose (after 48 hours)
Metabolic acidosis
  pH < 7.3
  Bicarbonate < 18 mmol/l
Encephalopathy
Renal failure
  Creatinine > 20 μmol/l
Coagulopathy
  INR > 3.0
Hypotension that does not respond to volume loading

Salicylate Overdose

ASSESSMENT

Plasma salicylate levels 4 hours after ingestion

The **features of salicylate toxicity** include:

Mild to **moderate**:
- Nausea and vomiting
- Tinnitus
- Hyperventilation
- Sweating
- Confusion

Severe
- Convulsions
- Coma

MANAGEMENT depends on plasma salicylate levels:

Under 45 mg/100 ml
   No treatment

45–65 mg/100 ml
   High fluid intake, intravenous route if necessary

Over 65 mg/100 ml
   Intravenous fluids
   Forced alkaline diuresis
   Medical referral

With significant overdoses the following investigations may be needed:

- Arterial blood: ABGs
- Venous blood:
   glucose, U&E
   prothrombin time
   FBC

Tricyclic Antidepressant Overdose

MANAGEMENT

Prevent further absorption of drug
Empty stomach if unconscious or if over 250 mg ingested

Activated charcoal 10–20 g orally

Anticipate and treat cardiac arrhythmias
12-lead ECG

Continuous ECG monitoring

Avoid anti-arrhythmic drugs except if in circulatory failure. Then use on a trial and error basis, either:
  Physostigmine salicylate 2 mg intravenous over 2 minutes
  Beta blockers
  Lignocaine

Treat convulsions
Diazepam by intravenous route

Chlormethiazole infusion

The following are of **no value**:
  Forced diuresis
  Haemodialysis
  Peritoneal dialysis

Organophosphate Poisoning

The clinical **FEATURES** include:

1. Acute **cholinergic syndrome** comprising;
   A peripheral **muscarinic** syndrome
   - Salivation
   - Lacrimation
   - Sweating
   - Diarrhoea
   - Miosis
   - Wheezing
   Nicotinic syndrome
   - Muscle fasciculation
   - Weakness
   - Convulsions
   - Coma
2. Non-cholinergic effects
   - Ventricular arrhythmias
   - Peripheral neuropathy

INITIAL MANAGEMENT

Check airway patency, adequacy of breathing and circulatory status

Decontaminate skin where indicated with thorough lavage with water

Take venous blood: cholinesterase

Atropinization
   Atropine 2 mg subcutaneously/intramuscularly/intravenously every 15–30 minutes until mouth dry and pupils dilated

Administer cholinesterase reactivator
   Pralidoxime

Solvent Abuse

A variety of substances are used for inhalation :

Adhesives
Corrector fluid
Gas lighter fuel
Nail varnish remover
Shoe polish and dyes
Dry cleaning fluids
Paint thinner/stripper
Hairspray
Furniture polish
Aerosol propellants
Deicer
Petrol

The usual **METHODS OF INHALATION** include:

- Soaked cloth (e.g. handkerchief)
- Plastic bag/crisp packet
- Direct from container

The **EFFECTS** are due to:

- Acute intoxication
- Asphyxiation
- Sudden death

The typical **STAGES OF INTOXICATION** mimic those of alcohol:

Initial **excitatory** phase with euphoria, disinhibition, disorientation, dizziness, tinnitus and hallucinations (visual and auditory)

Followed by **CNS depression**
Early: confusion, blurred vision, headache
Then: drowsiness, ataxia, dysarthria, nystagmus
Finally: seizures, loss of consciousness

The **user** is typically:

- Male
- Teenaged
- From low socioeconomic status

>

121

> Solvent Abuse

- Often ethnic minority
- From a disrupted family

The features of acute intoxication are:

- Rapid onset (within 2-3 minutes)
- Short duration
- No physical withdrawal symptoms

The **MANAGEMENT** is thus entirely supportive, taking care to ensure airway patency, adequate breathing and circulatory status.

The effects are self-limiting.

Button Battery Ingestion

The small size of button batteries makes them susceptible to be swallowed by inquisitive children.

MANAGEMENT of ingestion consists of the following steps:

Confirm ingestion
Plain X-rays of the abdomen and chest

Identify the type and make of battery used (with help from the Regional Poisons Unit)
Four types are generally available:

- Mercury cell
- Alkaline manganese cell
- Silver cell
- Lithium manganese dioxide cell

Determine the **position of the battery**

1. In the oesophagus
    Endoscopic removal is needed to prevent corrosion
2. In the stomach
    Observe radiologically by daily X-rays
    Cimetidine/ranitidine prevent gastric acid corrosion of battery case
3. Beyond the stomach
    If intact, observe
    If signs of corrosion and leakage, as evidenced by extravasation of radio-opaque battery contents on X-ray
    or if signs of peritoneal irritation
    or if signs of acute mercury poisoning (nausea and vomiting, increased salivation, personality change, tremor):
        Remove battery
        Check blood mercury level
        If level raised, mercury chelating agent, such as dimercaprol

Hallucinogenic Drug Overdose

These agents can be categorized as:

With SYMPATHOMIMETIC EFFECTS

Phenylethylamine derivatives (amphetamines)
  e.g. **Ecstasy (MDMA)**
Cocaine
Indole alkylamines
  Magic mushrooms: *Psilocybia*, *Gymnopilys* and *Panelous* genera
Peyote and Mescaline

With CHOLINERGIC EFFECTS

Muscimol and ibotenic acid containing mushrooms
  e.g. *Amanita muscaria* (Fly agaric)
    Amanita pantherina

LSD and **LSD-like compounds**

FEATURES OF OVERDOSE

Sympathomimetic
  Tremor
  Piloerection
  Tachycardia
  Increased blood pressure
  Dilated pupils

Psychedelic effects
Mood changes
  Euphoria
  Dysphoria
  Anxiety
  Panic
  Labile effect
  Paranoia

Perception disturbances
  Illusions: macropsia, micropsia, colour distortion, body image distortion
  Visual hallucinations, e.g. kaleidoscopic
  Synaesthesiae, e.g. seeing a smell, hearing a colour

Ecstasy

This is a popular name for 3,4-methylenedioxymethamphetamine, a synthetic amphetamine derivative.

It is taken orally as tablets or capsules containing 50–150 mg and is commonly available in night clubs and at raves.

The pharmacological effects of the drug may be compounded by physical exertion or dehydration.

Acute severe complications may lead to A&E attendance. The usual complications recorded include:

- Generalized shaking
- Jerking movements
- Convulsions
- Hypertension
- Tachycardia
- Hyperthermia
- Hypertonia
- Pupil dilatation

For **ACUTELY ILL** patients:

Check vital signs and core temperature
Rehydrate with intravenous fluids
Obtain 12-lead ECG and commence continuous monitoring
Control seizures with diazepam
Consider the need for
   Active cooling if hyperthermic
   Dantrolene
Refer to the medical team for admission
Notify the Regional Poisons Unit

Plant Poisoning

A variety of plants and their components may be ingested, usually accidentally, by both children and adults.

Useful information from the **HISTORY** includes:

Where was the plant growing?
- Field
- Roadside
- Garden
- Park
- Hedge

What was the appearance of the plant?
- Herb
- Shrub
- Tree

What parts were eaten?
- Fruits
- Leaves
- Roots

What was the size and colour of the fruits?

The patient or accompanying person may bring along the plant components, aiding identification. This may be aided by reference to illustrated books of plants or computerized databases.

GENERAL PRINCIPLES OF MANAGEMENT

Stabilize airway, breathing and circulation as needed

Consider naloxone or glucose if altered mentation

Empty the stomach if any doubt exists about the toxic nature of the plant, provided an acceptable time limit has elapsed following ingestion

Identify the plant

Consult Regional Poisons Unit

7 Gastrointestinal emergencies

Acute Abdominal Pain

The acute abdomen can often pose diagnostic problems in the A&E department. Following a systematic protocol is likely to minimize serious errors of omission.

It is important to characterize the pain as precisely as possible, concentrating on:

1. Site at onset and at present (either generalized, central, or in one or more quadrants)
2. Character (often patients find it difficult to describe pain in terms required of them by doctors), e.g.
   Steady, intermittent, colicky
3. Severity
4. Aggravating factors
   Movement
   Coughing
   Breathing
5. Relieving factors
   Lying still
   Specific posture
   Vomiting
   Food
   Drugs
6. Duration
7. Radiation, e.g.
   Shoulder tip
   Loin
   Groin
8. Progress
9. Associated symptoms
   Nausea and vomiting
   Anorexia
   Fever
   Faintness
   Jaundice
   Altered bowel habit
   Urinary symptoms
   Gynaecological symptoms

In all menstruating women the date of the last menstrual period should be ascertained.   >

INVESTIGATIONS

The role of investigations is limited as most common and significant causes of abdominal pain can be diagnosed clinically. A proportion of patients attending A&E will not have a clinically recognizable pattern of pain and examination and investigation can prove non-contributory. These patients comprise what is termed non-specific abdominal pain for the lack of a better term.

Urinalysis
  Cells
  Casts
  Blood

Venous blood
  FBC
  Amylase (levels > 1000 IU/l are diagnostic of acute pancreatitis)
  U&E (if vomiting)

Tests for pregnancy in all women of childbearing age

Plain X-ray of abdomen
  Limited value

Erect chest X-ray
  Gas under diaphragm with hollow viscus perforation

Ultrasound
  Gallstones
  Pancreatitis
  Abdominal aortic aneurysm

ACUTE APPENDICITIS

This is a common cause of the acute abdomen in A&E practice. Diagnosis is not always easy, particularly in the elderly and the very young, and where the location of the appendix is atypical, e.g. retrocaecal or pelvic.   >

> Acute Abdominal Pain

The use of a scoring system to add weight to the clinical diagnosis may be useful, such as the Alvarado Score:

	Score
Symptoms	
Migratory right iliac fossa pain	1
Anorexia	1
Nausea and vomiting	1
Signs	
Tenderness in the right iliac fossa	2
Rebound tenderness in the right iliac fossa	1
Elevated temperature	1
Laboratory findings	
Leucocytosis	2
Shift to the left of neutrophils	1
Total score	10

1–4 Unlikely
5–6 Possible
7–8 Probable appendicitis
9–10 Surgery needed

Acute appendicitis typically produces peritoneal irritation and the pain is aggravated by movement or by coughing, which is a useful pointer to the diagnosis.

A definitive diagnosis is often not possible, and surgical referral is indicated on clinical suspicion.

ACUTE ABDOMINAL PAIN WITH SHOCK

Faced with the signs of shock, the following possibilities must be considered:

Lesions causing **fluid loss**
    Acute pancreatitis
    Perforated peptic ulcer
    Mesenteric vascular occlusion
    Mechanical intestinal obstruction

>

> Acute Abdominal Pain

Lesions causing **blood loss**
  Ruptured abdominal aortic aneurysm
  Ruptured ectopic pregnancy
  Ruptured spleen or liver

Lesions with subsequent **sepsis**
  Perforated peptic ulcer
  Appendicitis with perforation
  Intestinal infarction
  Acute pelvic inflammatory disease

Acute Upper Gastrointestinal Bleeding

This can present with haematemesis and melaena or melaena alone.

The initial **ASSESSMENT** is to ascertain the severity of the bleed. Evaluation of this on the basis of observed external blood loss is unreliable. Haemodynamic stability, as judged on the basis of vital signs, is a useful objective marker of severity of bleeding, allowing categorization as follows:

Haemodynamically stable

Haemodynamically stable with signs of **compensation for blood volume deficit**

   Tachycardia

   Tachypnoea

Haemodynamically unstable

   Tachycardia

   Tachypnoea

   Hypotension, including postural fall in blood pressure

   Syncope

   Peripheral vasoconstriction

   Oliguria

Decompensated

   Confused

   Disoriented

   Weak, thready or absent peripheral pulses

   Unrecordable blood pressure

Initial **DOCUMENTATION** should include:

Vital signs (pulse rate, blood pressure, respiratory rate)

Skin: petechiae, bruising

Signs of **chronic liver disease**: ascites, jaundice, splenomegaly

Signs of **hepatocellular failure**: flapping tremor

Extent of **alcohol intake**

Medications especially aspirin and non-steroidal anti-inflammatory drugs (NSAIDs)

>

> Acute Upper Gastrointestinal Bleeding

Always check the nose and mouth for sources of bleeding which may lead to vomiting of swallowed blood.

ASSESSMENT and **RESUSCITATION** should proceed simultaneously

Two large-bore intravenous cannulae are sited in the ante-cubital fossae

Venous blood is taken for FBC, U&E, grouping and cross-matching (6 units if signs of volume depletion are present), prothrombin time and partial thromboplastin time

Volume replacement is commenced

Fresh frozen plasma and vitamin K 10 mg intravenously are given if a coagulation defect is identified

A urinary catheter is passed to commence hourly urine output monitoring

Patients over the age of 60 require a 12-lead ECG

A central venous pressure line may be needed if:

- The patient is shocked
- Is aged over 60
- Or has ischaemic heart disease

The patient is traditionally referred to the on-call medical team, who liaise with surgeons as appropriate

Early fibreoptic endoscopy is usually needed, within 12 hours of admission, to establish the source of blood loss

The common **CAUSES** of upper gastrointestinal bleeding include:

Oesophageal
Varices
Oesophagitis
Mallory-Weiss syndrome (oesophageal tear following violent emesis)

>

> Acute Upper Gastrointestinal Bleeding
Stomach and duodenum

Duodenal ulcer
Gastric ulcer
Gastritis: alcohol, NSAIDs
Acute stress ulceration
Neoplasia

Lower Gastrointestinal Bleeding

Initial **ASSESSMENT** includes:

Documentation of vital signs to ascertain haemodynamic
status

Characterizing the pattern of bleeding

Bright red blood is passed with brisk bleeding from any
source and from distal colorectal lesions

Slower bleeding of altered (darker red) blood mixed
with faeces with or without mucus indicates a

source in the proximal colon

Anorectal inspection may reveal haemorrhoids that have
prolapsed and ulcerated

Digital rectal examination and proctoscopy can be carried
out in A&E departments

MANAGEMENT

If the bleeding is profuse or producing haemodynamic
compromise, venous access and volume replacement
should be established. Surgical or medical referral is indicated depending on local arrangements.

For minor bleeding, investigation can be carried out on
an outpatient basis

Acute Anorectal Pain

The diagnosis of the cause can usually be made without difficulty from the history combined with anal inspection.

Formal rectal examination is often not possible owing to severe pain and sphincter spasm.

The usual **CAUSES** are:

Acute anal fissure
Hard stool (constipation)
Pain on and after defaecation
Blood-streaked stool

Perianal abscess
Severe constant throbbing pain
Sleep disturbance
Local induration and tenderness

Perianal haematoma
Painful swelling worsening over 24–48 hours, followed by gradual recovery
Localized swelling at anal verge, sometimes with a dark blue appearance caused by clot
If seen within 48 hours, incision and clot evacuation using local infiltration anaesthesia relieves the symptoms

Thrombosed, prolapsed or strangulated prolapsed internal haemorrhoids

Initial **management** is conservative, consisting of:
Bed rest
Local cold compresses
Topical local anaesthetic gels
Analgesics
Stool softeners if indicated
Severe symptoms may warrant hospitalization
Surgical evaluation is usually necessary for consideration of urgent haemorrhoidectomy

MANAGEMENT

Perianal haematoma: A&E
Anal fissure: GP initially   >

> Acute Anorectal Pain

Perianal abscess: surgical admission for incision and
  drainage (I&D) under general anaesthesia
Haemorrhoids with acute symptoms: surgical follow-up

Acute Diarrhoea

This can be defined as an increase in the frequency, fluidity and volume of stools. Most cases seen in A&E departments are suitable for treatment in the community.

ASSESSMENT

Number, volume and characteristics of stools
    Presence of blood
                mucus
Systemic symptoms, e.g. fever
Contacts with similar illness
Associated symptoms
    Vomiting
    Abdominal pain
    Tenesmus
Recent foreign travel
Recent meals away from home

CLINICAL ASSESSMENT includes:

State of hydration
    General appearance, e.g. lethargy, apathy, alertness
    Skin turgor
    Mucosal moistness
    Urine output
    Loss of weight

Vital signs
    Temperature
    Blood pressure
    Heart rate

INVESTIGATIONS

Venous blood
    U&E (only if clinically dehydrated)

Stool culture
    Only if:
        Recent foreign travel
        Institutionalized patient
        Patient a food handler

>

MANAGEMENT

Fluid replacement is the mainstay of treatment for acute
   infective diarrhoeas, which are generally self-limiting
   illnesses. This can be given orally if the patient is not
   vomiting

Antidiarrhoeal agents should not be used

Antiemetic agents should be used sparingly

Specific antimicrobial chemotherapy is rarely indicated:
   Severe *Campylobacter* infections
   Invasive salmonellosis (with systemic toxicity)
   Shigellosis

ORAL REHYDRATION SOLUTIONS

Composition (mmol/l)	Dextrolyte	Dioralyte	Rehidrat	WHO ORS
Na	35.0	35.0	50.0	90.0
K	13.4	20.0	20.0	25.0
Cl	30.5	37.0	50.0	80.0
Glucose	200.0	200.0	91.0	111.0
Sucrose	–	–	94.0	–
Bicarbonate	–	18.0	20.0	–
Citrate	–	–	9.0	10.0
Lactate	17.7	–	–	–
Osmolality	297	310	336	331

Acute Intestinal Obstruction

Assessment of the patient suspected of having an obstructed gut should aim to answer the following questions:

Is it really obstruction?

Colicky abdominal pain

Vomiting

Constipation or obstipation (inability to pass faeces or flatus)

Progressive abdominal distension

Not all of the above are necessary for a diagnosis but the presence of at least two is highly suggestive

Is strangulation of the gut likely?

Abdominal rigidity

Rebound tenderness

Irreducible hernia (inguinal, femoral, epigastric)

Systemic toxicity

What is the likely cause of obstruction?

The presence of laparotomy scars suggests adhesions as a possible cause

Rectal examination may suggest faecal impaction

Constipation and abdominal distension with inaudible or infrequent bowel sounds and no pain suggests paralytic ileus

What is the likely level of obstruction?

The higher the obstruction, the less the abdominal distension, and vomiting is more prominent as a symptom

Plain X-rays of the abdomen (supine) may help delineate the nature of the distended loops

Initial **INVESTIGATIONS** include:

Venous blood

FBC, U&E

X-rays of the abdomen

Erect (air–fluid levels; beware of acute gastroenteritis) >

> Acute Intestinal Obstruction

Supine (to show configuration of bowel loops distended)

MANAGEMENT

Obtain venous access with large-bore cannula

Commence volume replacement

Insert urethral catheter for continuous urine output measurement

Commence parenteral broad-spectrum antimicrobial therapy for suspected strangulation obstruction

Refer to the surgical team

Swallowed Foreign Bodies

X-rays to show the neck and chest at least are indicated if the foreign body or bodies ingested are likely to be radio-opaque. This confirms ingestion and the nature and position of the foreign bodies.

Oesophageal impaction often produces dysphagia with inability to swallow saliva, and localized discomfort. Urgent endoscopic removal is needed. Water-soluble contrast studies may be helpful to delineate the causative object, especially if radiolucent (e.g. dentures).

For objects in the **stomach**
    If **smooth**: watchful expectancy
    If **pointed**: consider endoscopic removal
For objects beyond the stomach
    If **smooth**: watchful expectancy
    If **pointed**: surgical removal if signs of gut perforation or intestinal obstruction

Acute oesophageal food impaction (Steakhouse Syndrome or Cafe Coronary) is usually seen in males. Predisposing factors include severe dental disease and poorly fitting dentures causing inadquate mastication of food boluses, and alcohol abuse.

Non-surgical removal may be possible, by using:
    An intravenous muscle relaxant, e.g. glucagon 1 mg and
    Effervescent granules (e.g. carbon dioxide producing granules) to distend the oesophagus

8 Gynaecological emergencies

Bleeding Per Vaginam

Check vital signs and look for clinical evidence of anaemia. Management depends on haemodynamic status and on whether or not pregnancy coexists.

Subsequent management depends on categorization of the patient into the following:

HAEMODYNAMICALLY UNSTABLE

Secure venous access with large-bore intravenous cannula
Take venous blood for FBC; group and save
Volume replacement
Gynaecological referral

HAEMODYNAMICALLY STABLE

Pregnancy test on urine or blood for beta subunit of human chorionic gonadotrophin (hCG)

If **PREGNANT**

Check Rhesus status; RhoGam is indicated
Abortion
Ectopic pregnancy
Antepartum haemorrhage

If **NON-PREGNANT**

Further assessment includes:
Length and interval of periods
Duration of excessive bleeding
Date of last menstrual period
Contraceptive technique
Hormonal therapy
Bimanual pelvic examination and speculum examination in presence of a chaperone
If no mass or ulcer, refer back to GP

Refer for gynaecological follow-up for all with
Postmenopausal bleeding
Bleeding associated with mass/ulcer

Abortion

Often leads to A&E attendance

Immediate management depends on haemodynamic status

The presence of signs of shock warrants setting up an intravenous line with a large-bore cannula, volume replacement, and grouping and cross-matching of blood.

If the patient is haemodynamically stable, a history and limited physical examination will help categorization into the following categories:

THREATENED

Bleeding per vaginam
No pain
Cervical os closed
Uterine size corresponds to calculated gestational age

INEVITABLE

Bleeding per vaginam
Pain
Dilating cervical os
Loss of clear fluid suggesting rupture of membranes

COMPLETE

Bleeding per vaginam slight and decreasing
No pain
Products of conception expelled

ADMISSION is needed in the following circumstances:

Threatened abortion
   High-risk pregnancy
   Precious pregnancy
   Difficulty coping at home
Inevitable abortion
Incomplete abortion

>

> Abortion

With all abortions, the Rhesus status of the patient must be ascertained if not already known. Rhesus-negative patients with Rhesus-positive partners need passive immunization with RhoGam within 72 hours of onset of bleeding.

With threatened abortion, an ultrasound scan may be advisable to confirm gestational age and confirm fetal viability.

Ectopic Pregnancy

This should be considered in the differential diagnosis of abdominal pain in any female of child-bearing age.

The menstrual history and subjective awareness of pregnancy may be unreliable. The presentation is often subtle and diagnosis often requires a high degree of clinical suspicion.

The **FEATURES** include:

Pain
> This is very variable in extent and character
> Shoulder tip pain represents irritation of the diaphragm by blood secondary to intraperitoneal rupture

A history of **menstrual abnormality** which may be either:
> A short period of amenorrhea (5–7 weeks) or
> A delayed period
> An abnormal period
> Non-cyclic bleeding

A normal menstrual history does not exclude ectopic pregnancy

Subjective symptoms of pregnancy such as:
> Morning sickness
> Breast tenderness
> Present in less than 50% of patients

With **RUPTURE** the presentation depends on the amount and rate of intraperitoneal bleeding:

1. **Massive intraperitoneal bleeding**
   > Severe abdominal pain
   > Pallor
   > Tachycardia
   > Hypotension
   > Peritonism
   > Cardiovascular collapse

2. **Slower intraperitoneal leakage of blood**
   > Lower abdominal pain, tenderness and guarding
   > Forniceal mass with tenderness

>

> Ectopic Pregnancy

HISTORY taking should include elucidation of possible
risk factors for ectopic pregnancy
Prior pelvic inflammatory disease
Presence of an intrauterine contraceptive device (IUCD)
Prior ectopic pregnancy
Prior tubal surgery for infertility
Infertility treatment, e.g. in vitro fertilization (IVF) or
gamete intra-fallopian transfer (GIFT)
Prior tubal ligation

Patients should be referred to a gynaecologist on suspicion. Pelvic examination is contraindicated if the diagnosis
is strongly suspected on clinical grounds.

When the patient presents with signs of acute massive
intraperitoneal rupture, the following should be done:
Two large-bore cannulae inserted to obtain venous
access
Venous blood for: FBC, group and cross-match
Urgent gynaecological referral

In all other situations an attempt must be made to prove
the presence of pregnancy by specific testing:
Urine pregnancy test: enzyme-linked immunoassay
(ICON) for beta subunit of hCG
Blood pregnancy test: radioimmunoassay for beta subunit of hCG

Acute Pelvic Inflammatory Disease

This is a cause of significant morbidity (particularly infertility) in women of childbearing age if inadequately assessed and treated. It should be considered in every woman of reproductive age who presents with lower abdominal pain. An adequate sexual, gynaecological or contraceptive history is essential.

The clinical **FEATURES** include:

Symptoms

- Bilateral lower abdominal pain
- Vaginal discharge
- Dysuria
- Deep dyspareunia
- Rectal discomfort
- Irregular menstrual bleeding
- Fever
- Low back pain

Signs

- Bilateral lower abdominal tenderness
- Rebound tenderness and guarding
- Adnexal masses
- Cervical excitation tenderness (pain on moving the cervix)
- Fever (temperature over 38°C)

RISK FACTORS that should be recorded in the history and which make the diagnosis more likely include:

Age under 25 years
Multiple sexual partners
Recent change of sexual partner
Previous episodes of pelvic inflammatory disease
Previous sexually transmitted disease
Current or recent use of IUCD
Recent pregnancy
Recent instrumentation of the uterus

>

> Acute Pelvic Inflammatory Disease

INVESTIGATIONS include:

FBC

Swabs: high vaginal
       endocervical
  including chlamydial swabs

Pregnancy test

INDICATIONS FOR ADMISSION

- Systemic toxicity
- Uncertain diagnosis
- Unable to tolerate treatment already prescribed
- Failure to respond to treatment
- Pelvic peritonitis

TREATMENT

Ensure proper follow-up after adequate microbiological specimens are obtained. The components of the multiple drug regimen include:

  Anti-chlamydial antibiotic
    Doxycycline 100 mg twice daily for 14 days
  Anaerobic infection
    Metronidazole 400 mg twice or thrice daily for 14 days
  Antigonococcal therapy (in selected instances)
    Ciprofloxacin 500 mg single dose

Partner investigation is mandatory (usually by a department of genitourinary medicine).

Postcoital Contraception

Generally this is the province of GPs and family planning clinics. Occasionally A&E departments may have to provide this service, particularly for rape victims and those at the latter part of the 72-hour period after unprotected coitus. Some departments may provide the service to all comers.

The general **INDICATIONS** are:

Unprotected intercourse
Contraceptive accidents e.g.
   Condom breakage or slippage
   IUCD expulsion
   Incorrect placement of diaphragm or cap
Missed pills
Sexual assault

The usual method provided in A&E is **hormonal**

This consists of the use of a combined oestrogen–progestogen pill. Schering PC4 (50 µg ethinyloestradiol and 50 µg norgestrel per tablet) is licensed for this purpose.

Two tablets should be taken as soon as possible, followed by two tablets 12 hours thereafter. The treatment is not effective over 72 hours after coitus. If the patient is on enzyme-inducing drugs (e.g. rifampicin) three tablets should be used instead of two.

If vomiting occurs within 3 hours of pill ingestion, the dose is repeated with an antiemetic (e.g. prochlorperazine). There is a failure rate of 2–3%.

In certain instances, presentation may be delayed beyond 72 hours. Emergency insertion of an IUCD may be effective up to 5 days after coitus.

Rape

The rape victim may occasionally attend A&E, largely as a result of physical injury.

Specific points to be noted in the **HISTORY** are:

- Time, date and place of occurrence
- Course of events
- Menstrual status
- Date of last menstrual period
- Normal sexual activity

MANAGEMENT is guided by whether or not this episode is being reported to the police

For the reporting victim, medical management must await the arrival of the police surgeon

For the non-reporting case, **ASSESSMENT** must be made of:

- Emotional state
- Physical injuries, both genital and extra-genital
- Genital trauma may warrant a gynaecological opinion
- Postcoital contraception may be required

Referral may be required to:
A Genitourinary Medicine Department (for prevention/ treatment of sexually transmitted disease)
Women's refuge
Criminal Injuries Compensation Board
Rape Crisis Centre
Victim Support Scheme

Follow-up and counselling is usually required.

9 Urological emergencies

Haematuria

The passage of blood per urethram is an alarming symptom which often leads to A&E attendance. Every episode of haematuria requires thorough investigation.

HISTORY taking should aim to elucidate the following:

Relationship of passage of blood to the urinary stream, which may be either:

Initial (from urethra or prostate)

Terminal (from bladder or posterior urethra)

Total (entire stream) (from upper urinary tract or from any cause of heavy haematuria)

The passage of clots signifies any source of heavy haematuria

Associated symptoms, which may originate from:

The lower urinary tract, e.g.

Frequency

Dysuria

Urgency

Suprapubic pain

Straining to void

Reduced calibre and force of urinary stream

The upper urinary tract, e.g.

Flank pain

Abdominal pain

Symptoms suggesting glomerular origin of bleeding

Ankle or facial swelling

Antecedent upper respiratory infection

Arthralgia

Medications

Anticoagulants (e.g. warfarin)

Cyclophosphamide

Past medical history

Renal stones

Diabetes mellitus

>

On **CLINICAL EXAMINATION**, the following should be looked for:

General
Pallor
Purpura
Oedema: face, sacral region, ankles
Vital signs: Pulse rate
blood pressure
temperature

Urinary tract
Tenderness in the loins or suprapubic region
Pelvic or abdominal mass
Rectal examination in men, feeling for the prostate
Genitalia, looking for any urethral meatal source of
bleeding

INVESTIGATIONS

Urine
Dipstick testing
Microscopy
To confirm presence or absence of red blood cells
This will help differentiate red urine due to pigments
Culture

Venous blood
FBC
U&E
Coagulation screen (if on warfarin)

X-ray
Intravenous urogram

All patients with frank haematuria need urological referral and follow-up in the absence of an identifiable glomerular source, in which case medical or nephrological follow-up is indicated.

Acute Ureteric Colic

This causes excruciatingly severe acute-onset unilateral loin pain, radiating both laterally and anteriorly, and distally to the groin and genitalia.

There is associated nausea and vomiting and restlessness, owing to the inability to find comfort in any position. A history of previous similar episodes may be obtained.

Associated symptoms that might be present include dysuria, discoloration of the urine, frank haematuria and the passage of solid material (gravel) via the urethra.

Initial assessment includes documentation of vital signs, noting temperature as well.

Abdominal examination often reveals renal angle tenderness. Beware of a leaking abdominal aortic aneurysm in the middle-aged or elderly patient.

MANAGEMENT

Provide prompt adequate **pain relief**, e.g. with diclofenac
    75 mg intramuscularly
Check urine by dipstick testing
Microscopic haematuria is present in 80% of patients
Send a specimen for culture
The investigation of choice is an **emergency intravenous urogram**, with films at 5, 10 and 20 minutes. If this is not carried out during the acute painful episode the calculus may be passed and the diagnosis will not be made.

The preliminary film may reveal a radio-opaque calculus within the line of the ureter. Plain films alone are unreliable. Phleboliths, calcified lymph nodes and vascular calcification may be difficult to distinguish from calculi.

If calculous disease is proven, the following investigations are ordered:
    Venous blood: U&E, creatinine, calcium
    Urine: calcium
    Stone analysis, where fragments are available
The patient must be referred for **urological follow-up >**

> Acute Ureteric Colic

ADMISSION is warranted if:

There is coexisting evidence of **infection** (fever)
If there is **persistent pain** in spite of adequate analgesia
If there is evidence of **persistent obstruction**

Acute Scrotal Pain

The cause varies according to the age of the patient:

Post-pubertal
Testicular torsion
Epididymo-orchitis
Torsion of testicular appendage
Trauma
Tumours with rapid growth

Pre-pubertal
Torsion of testicular appendage
Testicular torsion
Epididymo-orchitis
Idiopathic scrotal oedema
Trauma with haematocele formation

Neonates and infants
Testicular torsion
Epididymo-orchitis
Acute hydrocoele

TESTICULAR TORSION

Occurs mainly in children and adolescents

A history of prior self-limiting episodes may be present

Typically presents with acute-onset severe lower abdominal and scrotal pain, often accompanied by nausea and vomiting. Abdominal symptoms may predominate, drawing attention away from the testis. It is important that the external genitalia are examined in every instance of acute abdominal pain to avoid missing the diagnosis.

On **examination**, the following are found:
Markedly tender testis and epididymis
Abnormal lie of the testis
High in the scrotum with anterior epididymis
Absent cremasteric reflex

Urgent referral for surgical detorsion and orchidopexy is indicated.

>

ACUTE EPIDIDYMO-ORCHITIS

Presents with:

- Gradual onset of pain and swelling in the scrotum
- Dysuria and frequency of micturition
- Fever
- Urethral discharge
- Scrotal redness and oedema
- Spermatic cord thickening

Assessment includes urine dipstick testing for protein and blood, microscopy and culture

If it is difficult to feel the testis or a tumour is suspected, testicular ultrasound may help. Surgical advice should be sought in these circumstances

Urinary Tract Infections

Severe symptoms or systemic toxicity lead to A&E attendance. Based on the history, the following clinical syndromes can be recognized:

Cystitis
　　Frequency
　　Dysuria
　　Urgency
　　Suprapubic pain

Pyelonephritis
　　Frequency
　　Dysuria
　　Urgency
　　Fever
　　Loin pain

Prostatitis
　　Frequency
　　Dysuria
　　Urgency
　　Fever
　　Perineal, scrotal and back pain

Non-specific features may occur, specially in children:
　　Fever
　　Meningism
　　Diarrhoea and vomiting

PAST MEDICAL HISTORY may identify predisposing factors:

- Diabetes mellitus
- Renal disease
- Previous genitourinary abnormality or instrumentation

CLINICAL ASSESSMENT should include:

- Vital signs
- State of hydration
- Signs of systemic toxicity
- Urinalysis: dipstick testing
- Mid-stream urine for culture and sensitivity testing　　>

> Urinary Tract Infections

The results should be sent to the patient's GP to ensure adequate follow-up

FURTHER INVESTIGATION is necessary following the first urinary infection in all males, infants and children, and in females with:

- Frequent recurrences
- Persistent microscopic haematuria
- Persistent pyuria
- Acute pyelonephritis
- Associated hypertension
- Failure to respond to treatment

Acute Retention of Urine

Initial **ASSESSMENT**

Confirm that it is indeed retention and not oliguria
  Feel for suprapubic tenderness and fullness
  Percuss for suprapubic dullness

Confirm that spontaneous voiding is not possible
  Standing up, in privacy
  Warm baths may help

If this is not possible, urethral catheterization under aseptic conditions
  Use small gauge (14 or 16 Foley catheter), well lubricated, after instilling topical lignocaine gel in urethra

If the catheter is impassable, seek urological assistance
  Suprapublc cystotomy is usually needed

After relief of acute symptoms:
  Check for palpable urethral stricture
  Assess for: perianal painful lesions
               perineal bruising or swelling
  Perform rectal examination with bladder empty. This may reveal faecal impaction or a large prostate (although this has little correlation with the degree of urinary obstruction)

If preceding symptoms suggest prostatism, i.e. reduced stream calibre and force, increased night frequency of micturition, refer for urological follow-up, with catheter retained in situ.

If this episode is due to drugs or a painful local lesion, a trial of voiding without the catheter should be made.

Always send the urine obtained for dipstick testing, microscopy and culture.

10 Rheumatological emergencies

Back Pain

This may be a reason for A&E attendance in the following circumstances:

- Acute onset, with or without preceding trauma
- Severe intractable pain
- Second opinion for pain already being treated by GP
- Neurological symptoms
- Systemic symptoms

On the basis of the history, back pain can be categorized into one of the following groups:

Mechanical
Worsened by movement
Worse on prolonged sitting or standing
Relieved by rest

Inflammatory
Associated with morning stiffness
Often relieved by exercise

Neurological
Root radiation, including girdle pain
Neurological signs (including bowel and bladder symptoms)

Sinister (neoplasm or bone sepsis)
Recent onset
Systemic symptoms and signs
Fever
Weight loss
Pain at rest
Sleep disturbance
Localized marked tenderness
Coexisting or previous recent malignancy

ASSESSMENT includes:

Gait
Stance
Straight leg raising in both legs

>

Spinal deformity
  Loss of lumbar lordosis
  Scoliosis
Localization of tenderness
  Spinous process
  Paraspinal

Neurological assessment

Muscle power
  L2 Hip flexion (iliopsoas)
  L3–L4 Knee extension (quadriceps)
  L4 Ankle dorsiflexion (tibialis anterior)
  L5 Great toe extension (extensor hallucis longus)
  S1–S2 Knee flexion (hamstrings)
          Ankle plantarflexion (gastrocnemius)
          Buttock contraction (glutei)

Sensation in dermatomes
  L4 Medial knee
  L5 Lateral calf and great toe
  S1 Lateral foot and little toe
  S2–S4 Perianal and perineal regions

Reflexes
  L3, L4 Knee jerk
  S1   Ankle jerk

Rectal examination for sphincter tone

Abdominal examination for aortic aneurysm

Examination of testicles for possible tumour

INVESTIGATIONS

Lumbar spine X-rays are of little or no value in acute non-traumatic back pain

Findings are often incidental and may not adequately explain the current episode of pain, such as:

● Localized degenerative changes
● Disc space narrowing
● Disc calcification

>

- Spondylosis
- Spina bifida occulta
- Schmorl's nodes

Oblique views are required to visualize facet joints if necessary

Screening tests for inflammatory, metabolic or neoplastic causes

FBC
ESR/plasma viscosity
Calcium
Alkaline phosphatase
Acid phosphatase
Protein electrophoresis
Bone scan

Specific tests for disc prolapse

Myelography
CT/MRI scan

A condition to beware of is **central disc prolapse**
This is a neurosurgical emergency
The features include:

- Acute low back pain
- Bilateral lower limb symptoms
  Paraesthesiae
  Numbness
- Saddle anaesthesia
- Urinary retention
- Constipation

ACUTE LUMBAR DISC PROLAPSE

This condition is overdiagnosed as a cause of acute low back pain. The diagnosis on clinical grounds requires the following features:

Nerve root symptoms

Unilateral leg pain which is the dominant complaint rather than back pain

>

Paraesthesiae or numbness in a dermatome distribution
- L4: medial leg
- L5: lateral calf and/or dorsum of foot
- S1: lateral foot and sole

Nerve root irritation signs
Straight leg raising less than 50% of normal reproducing leg pain

Pain reproduced by raising uninvolved leg (crossover pain)

Nerve root compression signs
Weakness

Sensory loss in dermatome

Loss of or impaired reflexes

Postural deformities of lumbar spine
Lateral scoliotic tilt

Obliteration of lordosis

Acutely Painful Joint

The usual **CAUSES** can be categorized as:

In a previously normal joint

Crystal-induced arthritis (gout, pseudogout)
Septic arthritis
Trauma
Traumatic synovitis
Haemarthrosis

In a previously damaged joint

Exacerbation of underlying disease (osteoarthritis, rheumatoid arthritis)
Septic arthritis

ASSESSMENT includes:

- Possible precipitating factors
Blunt or penetrating trauma
- Features related to the joint
Pain
Tenderness
Swelling
Redness
Heat
- State of other joints
- Systemic features
Temperature
Toxicity
- Extra-articular features
Gouty tophi
- Evidence of other disease
Diabetes mellitus

Investigations useful in the elucidation of the cause
VENOUS BLOOD: **FBC**

Acute phase reactants (e.g. C Reactive Protein)
Culture (suspected sepsis)

>

> Acutely Painful Joint

SYNOVIAL FLUID: Aspiration under aseptic conditions
Microscopy for pus cells
Polarising light microscopy for
crystals
Gram stain
Culture and sensitivity testing

X-RAYS: of the joint in AP & lateral planes

Features suggesting septic arthritis

Rapid progression

Fever

Systemic toxicity

Marked periarticular muscle spasm with gross limitation of joint movement

Local cellulitis

Regional lymphadenopathy

Risk factors for septic arthritis
Local factors

Penetrating trauma

Intravenous drug abuse

Joint prosthesis

Systemic factors

Immunosuppressive therapy

Steroids

Cytotoxic drugs

Diabetes mellitus

Sickle cell disease

Alcohol abuse

Management of septic arthritis

Refer to orthopaedic surgeon or rheumatologist for admission

Acute Calf Pain

This not uncommon symptom is often regarded as one with a possibly sinister cause. The main consideration is to exclude the possibility of deep vein thrombosis which usually warrants admission and anticoagulation.

Initial **ASSESSMENT** should concentrate on the relation of the symptom to preceding trauma

If pain immediately followed **direct** or **indirect trauma** it is likely to be due to either:

1. Tear of the calf muscles (gastrocnemius/soleus)
   Sudden onset
   Tenderness related to medial head of gastrocnemius
   Pain worsened by stretching calf muscles (passive ankle dorsiflexion)
   Delayed onset of bruising around the malleoli of the ankle

2. A contusion of the calf muscles

In the absence of trauma the following possibilities should be considered:

Deep vein thrombosis
Ruptured popliteal cyst
   Popliteal swelling with knee fully extended
   Knee joint effusion
Cellulitis
   Redness
   Brawny induration
   Fever

In considering the diagnosis of deep vein thrombosis it must be remembered that signs and symptoms are non-specific.

As part of the routine, questioning should be directed to ascertain the presence of **risk factors for thrombo-embolic disease:**

- Previous thromboembolism
- Obesity   >

> Acute Calf Pain

- Malignancy
- Pregnancy and puerperium
- Oral contraception (high oestrogen)
- Varicose veins
- Trauma or orthopaedic surgery to the pelvis or lower limbs recently
- Haematological disorders with thrombotic tendency
- Age over 60 years
- Immobility

A clinical suspicion of deep vein thrombosis always requires radiological confirmation, by either duplex ultrasound or contrast venography before admission and anticoagulation.

Acute Shoulder Pain

LIKELY CAUSES

Calcific supraspinatus tendinitis
Rotator cuff sprain
                tear: partial
                         complete
Frozen shoulder (adhesive capsulitis)
Glenohumeral joint arthritis
Referred pain

ASSESSMENT

History of trauma
Specific symptoms
    Pain
    Stiffness
    Sleep disturbance
    Swelling
Symptoms elsewhere
    Neck
    Cardiac
    Respiratory
Past medical history

FROZEN SHOULDER

Features

    Painful restriction of passive and active shoulder movements
    Night pain with sleep loss
    Diffuse anterior shoulder tenderness
    Wasting of deltoid and supraspinatus muscles

Predisposing factors

    Shoulder trauma
    Neurological disease leading to hemiplegia
    Cardiac disease and surgery
    Diabetes mellitus

>

ACUTE CALCIFIC SUPRASPINATUS TENDINITIS

Features

Acute onset of localized shoulder pain
No preceding trauma
  Sleep disturbance
  Maximal tenderness in region of supraspinatus attachment to greater tuberosity of humerus
  Calcific deposit on X-ray

Acute Wrist Pain

INITIAL ASSESSMENT comprises noting the following:

History of preceding trauma and, if so, mechanism
Hand dominance
Overuse or unaccustomed activity at work or recreation
Relation to activity and rest
Prior episodes of pain and treatment thereof
Associated symptoms
  Swelling
  Stiffness
  Creaking on movement (crepitus)

On **EXAMINATION**, the following should be noted:

Look
  Swelling
  Deformity
  Skin changes: rednesss, bruising

Feel
  Localized tenderness
  Crepitus on passive movement
  Swelling, including ganglia on dorsal aspect
  Finkelstein's test: passive wrist ulnar deviation with
    thumb adducted causes pain in the presence of De
    Quervain's disease [tenosynovitis of abductor pollicis
    longus (APL) and extensor pollicis brevis (EPB)
    tendons]
  Sensation in hand (particularly median nerve distribu-
    tion)
  Radial pulse

Move
  Wrist dorsiflexion and palmar flexion
    Ulnar and radial deviation
  X-rays may be needed if bony trauma is likely, e.g.
    Deformity
    Local bony tenderness with swelling

>

MANAGEMENT depends on the cause and may include:

- Rest in wrist splint or POP slab or cast
- Non-steroidal anti-inflammatory agents
- Injection of steroid and local anaesthetic

11 Geriatric emergencies

Assessment of the Elderly

With a steadily increasing elderly population, often with multiple symptoms and on multiple medications, A&E attendance may often result from a complex interplay between medical and social factors.

Systematic assessment of the elderly is important before the decision to send home is made.
The following should be documented in all patients except where the attendance is for trivial self-limiting illness or injury.

Mental state
Alert/apathetic/confused
Mobility: unaided/with assistance/unable

Vision

Hearing

Dentition

Continence

Personal items
Hearing aids
Dentures
Walking aids (e.g. stick, Zimmer frame)
Spectacles

Housing
House: own/council/rented
Flat: ground floor/upper (lift?)
Bungalow: own/council
Sheltered housing: resident warden
Residential accommodation: local authority/private/voluntary

Lives with
Spouse
Family member
Friend
Other
Alone

>

Activities of self care
　Washing
　Feeding
　Dressing
　Toileting

Current medication
　Supervision of drug therapy at home by:
　　Relative
　　Neighbour
　　District nurse
　　Health visitor
　　Home help

Daily support or services
　Family member
　Neighbour
　Friend
　Home help
　Meals on wheels

The **abbreviated mental test score** allows objective evaluation of mental state:
　Age
　Time
　Address for recall at end of test
　Year
　Name of hospital
　Recognition of two persons
　Date of birth
　Name of present monarch
　Count backwards from 20 to 1
　Year of First World War

Community Services for the Elderly

Awareness of what is available in the community may help in the coordination of safe discharge of the elderly patient from the A&E department.

SOCIAL SERVICES DEPARTMENT

Home help
Meals on wheels (initially set up by the WRVS)
Night sitter
Day centre
Social worker
Residential home
Holiday admission (respite care)

COMMUNITY NURSING

District Nurse
Bath attendant
Tuck-in service
Specialist nurses
    Diabetic
    Incontinence
    Community psychiatric
    Terminal care

COMMUNITY PHYSIOTHERAPY

Falls in the Elderly

Falls in the elderly often lead to them being brought to an A&E. This occurs not only following falls in public places, but also in residential institutions and at home. The purpose of the visit is often to ascertain not only the cause of the fall but to identify any complications of the fall, and injury in particular. The cause of falls is often multifactorial and may be symptomatic of unrecognized physical illness.

FACTORS LEADING TO FALLS IN THE ELDERLY:

Environmental hazards
Uneven paving
Steps
Slippery floors
Wires
Objects on the floor
Poor lighting

Intrinsic factors

1. **Defective sensory input**
   Visual impairment
   Dizziness due to vestibular disorder
   Peripheral neuropathy with loss of position sense

2. **Disorders of gait**
   Cerebellar ataxia
   Spasticity
   Parkinsonism

3. **Disorders of the central nervous system**
   Epileptic seizures
   Transient ischaemic attacks

4. **Cardiovascular disorders**
   Cardiac arrhythmias
   Postural hypotension
   Effort syncope

5. **Musculosketal disorders**
   Arthritis with joint stiffness

>

> **Falls in the Elderly**

    Unstable joints
    Myopathy, e.g. due to osteomalacia

6. **Alcohol abuse**

7. **Drop attacks**

The basic minimal **ASSESSMENT** after a fall includes the following:

1. **History**
    Circumstances of the fall, including:
      Environmental hazards, posture change, head turning or other activity
    Associated symptoms, such as dizziness, fainting, palpitations, chest pain

2. **General examination**
    Mental state
    Gait
    Vision
    Hearing

3. **Drug history**
    Sedatives, tranquillizers, hypnotics, alcohol, anti-hypertensive therapy, diuretics

4. Supine and standing blood pressure

5. Evidence of:
    Cardiac arrhythmia
    Muscle weakness, rigidity or tremor
    Injury to head, face, trunk or limbs
    Arthritis
    Foot deformities

6. Mobility, with or without assistance

A useful way to categorize the patient who has **REPEATED UNEXPLAINED FALLS** follows:

Consciousness impaired

1. **Postural**
    Postural hypotension
    Micturition syncope

>

2. **Non-postural**

    Transient ischaemic attack
    Epileptic seizure
    Cardiogenic episodes
        Stokes-Adams' attacks
        Aortic stenosis

Consciousness unimpaired

    Drop attacks

Acute Confusional State

Acute onset of confusional states is a frequent response in the older individual to a variety of systemic disturbances which are amenable to treatment, implying that this is often a reversible condition.

The typical **FEATURES** include:

Clouding of consciousness
Fluctuation in the level of consciousness, with an altered
    sleep–wake cycle
Disorientation in time and place
Altered perception, with illusions , misinterpretations and
    hallucinations
Disorganized thought
Impairment of memory (registration, recall and retention)
Motor overactivity, with restlessness
Emotional changes, such as anxiety, panic and terror
The symptoms are usually worse at night

Initial **ASSESSMENT** includes:

Level of consciousness
Mini-mental test score
Vital signs
State of hydration
Physical examination of the cardiovascular, respiratory
    and neurological systems
Examination of the abdomen
Medication history
Past medical history
Alcohol intake history
Signs of trauma, particularly to the head

Initial **INVESTIGATIONS** include:

Urine dipstick testing for blood and protein, followed
    by microscopy and culture where these prove to be
    positive
Venous blood: glucose, U&E, FBC
                LFT, thyroid function (where indicated)

>

Chest X-ray
12-lead ECG

A list of the **CAUSES** is useful as a checklist in helping
to make the diagnosis:

Dehydration
Infections
  Chest
  Urinary tract
  Septicaemia
Intoxication or withdrawal
  Alcohol
  Prescribed medication
Heart failure, myocardial infarction
Intracranial lesions
  Subdural haematoma
  Tumours
  Infection, especially meningitis
  Cerebrovascular accident
  Post-ictal phase of epilepsy
Respiratory failure
Carcinomatosis
Metabolic disorders
  Liver failure
  Renal failure
Endocrine disorder
  Hypoglycaemia
  Hypothyroidism/hyperthyroidism

MANAGEMENT
Referral to the on-call medical team for admission is indi-
cated. Be certain that this is acute confusion and not a
long-standing dementia.
Specific management is for the underlying cause
Supportive management includes reassurance
  Occasionally sedation may be required for agitation,
    with haloperidol or a phenothiazine.

Gone Off Feet

The elderly person who is unable to walk may be brought into the A&E department for assessment, particularly when this is impairing care at home or in residential accommodation.

Often the deterioration is gradual and multifactorial, with no clear history of preceding trauma.

Under these circumstances a thorough examination of all body systems is necessary, taking into account the fact that any of the following situations may lead to the presentation with immobility:

1. **Cardiorespiratory problems**
   Shortness of breath on exertion
   Intermittent claudication

2. **Neurological problems**
   Peripheral neuropathy
   Parkinsonism
   Unsuspected cerebrovascular accident

3. **Generalized weakness**
   Electrolyte abnormalities
      Hyponatraemia
      Hypokalaemia
   Myopathy
      Osteomalacia
      Malignancy

4. **Painful feet**
   e.g. due to long toe nails

5. **Recent fall(s)** leading to loss of confidence

6. **Psychiatric problems**
   Dementia
   Depression

7. **Unsuspected lower limb fractures**, particularly of the femoral neck

12 Environmental emergencies

Near Drowning

The **factors that predispose to submersion accidents** include:

Alcohol abuse

Psychomotor depressive drugs

Injury, e.g. cervical spine trauma following diving accidents

Convulsions

Myocardial infarction

Cerebrovascular accident

Poor swimming ability

Hypoglycaemia

Child abuse

Attempted suicide

MANAGEMENT depends on clinical state of the patient

In cardiac arrest

Commence CPR

Continue resuscitation until rewarming complete

Conscious on arrival

Not hypoxic, received mouth to mouth resuscitation

Admit for 48 hours

Correct hypothermia (temperature under 35°C)
metabolic acidosis (pH < 7.2)

Observe for late-onset cerebral oedema and pulmonary oedema

Hypoxic: aspirated water: breathing spontaneously

Admit

Correct hypoxia
hypothermia
metabolic acidosis

Antibiotics if contaminated water or sewage aspirated

Steroids

Hypoxic: aspirated water: inadequate spontaneous ventilation

Intubate and ventilate

Admit to Intensive Therapy Unit (ITU)   >

> Near Drowning

Correct hypovolaemia
Monitor central venous pressure (CVP)

All conscious patients should receive the following
ASSESSMENT:

- Airway patency
- Adequacy of breathing
- Vital signs, including temperature with low-reading rectal thermometer
- Pulse oximetry
- X-rays of the chest and cervical spine
- Venous blood: U&E
- Arterial blood: ABGs
- ECG monitoring

POSSIBLE EFFECTS OF DROWNING include:

Dry drowning

Caused by reflex laryngospasm leading to asphyxiation

Wet drowning

Leading to widespread atelectasis, pulmonary oedema, gross ventilation/perfusion mismatch, surfactant depletion and reduced lung compliance

Fresh or salt water probably do not make much difference to the outcome

Immersion syndrome

Sudden death from cardiac arrest caused by very cold water contact

Secondary drowning

Aspiration pneumonia developing 48-72 hours later

Cold Injury

Apart from the risk of hypothermia, low environmental temperatures can lead to frostbite.

Contributory factors include:

- Wind velocity
- Moisture
- Lack of adequate clothing
- Use of alcohol

Initial **ASSESSMENT** includes:

- Appearance of the area: colour

    bullae
- Sensation
- Capillary refill after blanching
- Temperature
- Oedema

MANAGEMENT

For injuries where tissue viability is impaired, admission to hospital is required. The principles of treatment include:

Rapid thawing by immersion of the affected part in a water bath (at a temperature of 40–42°C)

Thawing is continued until the area is soft, red and sensate.

Adjuncts to treatment include:

Intravenous analgesia

Tetanus immunization

Low molecular weight dextran

Heparin

Careful handling of the affected area

Hypothermia

Hypothermia is diagnosed when the core temperature of the body falls below 35°C.

It can be classed according to severity as:

- Mild: 35–34°C
- Moderate: 34–30°C
- Severe < 30°C

The immediate causative factor is **cold exposure**
Contributory factors include the following:

Socio-economic
Low room temperature due to inadequate heating

Drugs
Alcohol
Major tranquillizers (phenothiazines)

Illness
Dementia
Metabolic/endocrine disorders
Diabetes mellitus
Myxoedema
Immobility
Neurological disorder, e.g. cerebrovascular accident
Severe arthritis

ASSESSMENT AND MANAGEMENT

Confirm the diagnosis with a low-reading rectal thermometer in the empty rectum
Administer 60% oxygen by face mask
Establish venous access
At the same time obtain venous blood for FBC, U&E, glucose, amylase
Pulse oximetry
12-lead ECG, followed by continuous ECG monitoring
Commence slow **passive rewarming** with metallic insulating space blankets
Aim at a rise of 0.5°C per hour

>

> Hypothermia

Minimal and gentle handling to avoid precipitating ventricular fibrillation

Active external rewarming should be avoided, as it can result in:

Cardiovascular collapse from compartmental fluid shifts

After drop: a paradoxical drop in core temperature with rewarming

Cardiac arrhythmias, particularly ventricular fibrillation

In severe hypothermia, active core rewarming may be needed, e.g. by heated pleural or peritoneal lavage, or cardiopulmonary bypass.

All patients should be referred to the medical on-call team.

Carbon Monoxide Poisoning

Acute heavy exposure to carbon monoxide can result from:

- Poorly ventilated heating systems
- Exposure to car exhaust fumes, in a closed car or garage
- Methylene chloride inhalation (from paint stripper)

The symptoms are variable, non-specific and can be misleading if a clear history of environmental exposure is not obtained. Carbon monoxide poisoning must be considered in the differential diagnosis of unexplained coma, in which case carboxyhaemoglobin estimation may be helpful.

Typical symptoms include:

- Headache
- Dizziness
- Blurred vision
- Confusion
- Nausea and vomiting
- Convulsions
- Coma

MANAGEMENT IN A&E

100% oxygen via oronasal mask
Venous blood carboxyhaemoglobin on arrival
Arterial blood gases
Consideration of the need for
   Artificial ventilation
   or
   Hyperbaric oxygen therapy
12-lead ECG

Be aware of the possibility of deliberate self-harm, which may need to be assessed after treatment of the acute phase

Pulse oximetry is unreliable in the presence of carboxy-haemoglobin

>

> Carbon Monoxide Poisoning

Hyperbaric oxygen may be needed if:

- The patient is unconscious
- Neurological signs are present
- Cardiac complications occur
- Carboxyhaemoglobin levels are above 40%
- The patient is pregnant

All serious carbon monoxide poisoning cases should be discussed with the local hyperbaric therapy unit.

Dog Bites

ASSESSMENT

- Mechanism
- Circumstances of attack: provoked/unprovoked
- Breed of dog where known
- Risk of rabies (if bitten in foreign country)
- Tetanus immunization status

INJURY PATTERNS

- Puncture wounds
- Abrasions
- Lacerations
- Flap lacerations
- Tissue loss

MANAGEMENT

Clean thoroughly with saline

Primary skin closure for facial injuries

Delayed skin closure for limb injuries that require closure (at 72 hours)

Broad-spectrum antibiotics

Tetanus prophylaxis

Rabies vaccination where indicated (advice from the Central Public Health Service Laboratory in Colindale is available)

Refer to plastic surgeon where complicated by tissue loss

Adder Bites

The adder (*Vipera berus*) is the only poisonous snake in the British Isles.

With suspected or proven adder bite:

- Reassure the patient
- Clean and dress the wound(s)
- Keep the involved limb dependent
- **Admit** to hospital for 24 hours for observation, which consists of:
    Hourly pulse rate and blood pressure
    Urine output monitoring
    Serial limb girth measurement
    12-lead ECG twice daily
    ECG monitoring if hypotensive
    Coagulation screen if bleeding
       Baseline FBC, U&E

Zagreb **antivenom** is indicated for:

- Hypotension
- Bleeding
- ECG changes
- Leucocytosis > 20 000/mm^3

ADMINISTRATION

Two ampoules of antivenom are diluted to 100 ml with normal saline and administered at the rate of 15 drops per minute via an intravenous infusion

13   Metabolic/endocrine emergencies

Hypoglycaemia

This is a frequent cause of A&E attendance, particularly in insulin-dependent diabetics, and is rarely due to other causes.

Recurrent attendances because of hypoglycaemia warrant medical referral.

Hypoglycaemia is defined as a plasma glucose < 2.5 mmol/l irrespective of symptoms.

FEATURES OF HYPOGLYCAEMIA

Early warning symptoms

All diabetics should be familiar with these symptoms as part of a patient education programme:

Circumoral tingling

Sweating

Hunger

Tremulousness

Palpitations

Early morning headache (with nocturnal hypoglycaemia)

Established hypoglycaemia consists of varying combinations of the following symptoms and signs:

Neuroglycopenic

Mild: Double vision

Difficulty in concentration

Dysarthria

Moderate: Confusion

Behaviour change

Late: Restlessness

Seizures

Focal neurological signs, e.g. hemiparesis

Coma

Decerebrate rigidity

Adrenergic

Sweating

Palpitations

Tremor

Pallor

>

Tachycardia
Anxiety
Mydriasis

TREATMENT

Once recognized, aided by a BM Stix determination on finger prick blood (a venous blood sample for plasma glucose is advisable for confirmation), treatment should be prompt to avoid cerebral damage.

If the patient is able to swallow, 10–20g of oral simple (rapidly absorbed) carbohydrate is given, e.g.
Sugar, 2 teaspoonfuls
Sugar lumps, 3 small lumps
Lucozade, 60 ml
Ribena, 15 ml

If the patient is unable to swallow, IV 50 ml 50% dextrose (25 g glucose) is given in an antecubital vein taking care to avoid extravasation
If venous access is difficult, 1 mg glucagon may be given subcutaneously or intramuscularly.
Twenty minutes should be allowed for action and the injection should not be repeated. Glucagon is particularly useful in pre-hospital situations.

In the patient who has recovered, and particularly with repeated recent episodes, an attempt must be made to ascertain the cause for the hypoglycaemic episode.

The likely causes include:

Altered eating patterns
Missing meals
Reducing meals
Delaying meals

Altered exercise patterns
Excessive exercise
Unaccustomed exercise

Alcohol abuse   >

> Hypoglycaemia

Reduced insulin requirements
  e.g. change to human insulin

Too much insulin

Altered awareness of hypoglycaemia, e.g. human insulin, beta blockers

Other drugs potentiating oral hypoglycaemics

Diabetic Ketoacidosis

This is a life-threatening emergency, which is usually easy to diagnose, especially when occurring in previously diagnosed diabetics. Occasionally it may be the presenting feature in undiagnosed diabetics. It should be suspected whenever the condition of an insulin-dependent diabetic deteriorates.

CLINICAL FEATURES

Severe **dehydration**, due to osmotic diuresis, vomiting, diarrhoea, hyperventilation and fever
The usual fluid deficit on arrival in hospital ranges between 5 and 10 litres
Ketosis, with hyperventilation due to metabolic acidosis (Kussmaul's breathing)
Gastrointestinal symptoms
  Nausea and vomiting
  Acute abdominal pain which may mimic a surgical abdomen
  Paralytic ileus
Depressed level of consciousness
Signs of **shock**

INVESTIGATION AND MANAGEMENT should proceed simultaneously. Early medical or paediatric referral is mandatory
  Commence an intravenous infusion using a large-bore cannula
    Normal saline is used to replace fluid deficit
    1st 15 minutes: 500 ml
    Then 1 litre over 1 hour for first 4 hours
  Commence insulin infusion
    Attach an infusion pump by a four-way tap to the intravenous line
    24 units Actrapid insulin are made up to 20 ml with normal saline in a plastic syringe
    The administration rate is 6–8 units (0.1 units/kg/hour) hourly

>

> Diabetic Ketoacidosis

Commence ECG monitoring

Avoid oral intake initially because of coexisting ileus

Pass a nasogastric tube if ileus present or gag reflex is impaired

Consider use of antibiotics

Monitor blood glucose and U&E hourly

Give colloid (e.g. Haemaccel) if persistently hypotensive or oliguric with above regime

Replace potassium after the first hour, guided by serum levels (hopefully, the patient will no longer be in A&E by this time)

Level (mmol /l)	Administration rate (mmol/hr)
3.5	40
3.5–4.0	30
4.0–5.0	20
5.0	Nil

No potassium should be given if the patient is anuric

ASSESSMENT OF THE KETOACIDOTIC PATIENT

Severity

Venous blood

Glucose

U&E

FBC

Ketones

Arterial blood: ABGs

Plasma osmolarity

Possible precipitating cause

Physical examination

Chest X-ray

Blood culture

Urine microscopy and culture

Non-Ketotic Hyperglycaemic Coma

The clinical **FEATURES** include:

- A predilection for elderly individuals with type II (non-insulin-dependent) diabetes mellitus, which is often previously undiagnosed.
- The onset is insidious
- The presentation is with confusion or coma
- Severe dehydration is usually present
- Ketosis is minimal or absent
- Severe hyperglycaemia (blood glucose over 50 mmol/l) is usual
- Polyuria and polydipsia are present. The use of glucose-containing drinks (e.g. Cola, Lucozade) to quench the ensuing thirst is often an aggravating factor
- Reversible focal neurological deficits may occur
- Thromboembolic events (cerebral, pulmonary and mesenteric) can complicate the condition. Heparinization is thus usually recommended.

INVESTIGATIONS

Venous blood glucose; U&E, **plasma osmolality**

Can be calculated from formula $2 \times (Na+K) +$ glucose + urea giving a figure in mosmol/kg. This is usually greater than 350 mosmol/l

12-lead ECG

MANAGEMENT

This follows the general scheme as suggested for keto-acidosis. The differences are:

If the serum sodium is over 150 mmol/l, half strength (0.45%) saline should be used in place of normal (0.9%) saline.

The insulin infusion rate can be slower (at 3 units/hour)
Medical referral is indicated

Hyperkalaemia

A potentially life-threatening situation can arise from high levels of serum potassium, determined on a non-haemolysed venous blood sample.

Initial **INVESTIGATIONS**:

- Venous blood: U&E
- 12-lead ECG

MANAGEMENT

Stop any potassium-containing intravenous infusion
Reverse membrane effects
    10–30 ml 10% calcium gluconate slow intravenously over 10 minutes
Encourage intracellular translocation of potassium
    8.4% sodium bicarbonate
    10% dextrose with 20 units Actrapid insulin per 100 g Glucose as an intravenous infusion
Remove potassium from the body
    Potassium exchange resin
      Kayexalate 20–30 g orally
    Loop diuretics, e.g. frusemide
    Dialysis
Continuous ECG monitoring
Monitor serum potassium level

Addisonian Crisis (Acute Adrenal Insufficiency)

This life-threatening condition can be secondary to one of the following situations:

- Stress in the presence of chronic adrenocortical insufficiency where steroid requirements are not adequately replaced, e.g. trauma, infection, surgery
- Acute bilateral adrenocortical haemorrhage complicating septicaemia, e.g. meningococcaemia
- Abrupt stoppage of long-term steroid therapy

The **FEATURES** include:

- Hypotension
- Cardiovascular collapse
- Nausea and vomiting
- Abdominal pain
- Fever
- Confusion

INVESTIGATIONS

Venous blood: U&E, glucose, calcium, FBC

Typical findings include: hyponatraemia
hyperkalaemia
hypoglycaemia
azotaemia

MANAGEMENT

Commence treatment on clinical suspicion
Venous access with large-bore cannula
Commence normal (0.9%) saline
Hydrocortisone 200 mg intravenously
Treat hypoglycaemia with 50% dextrose intravenously
Refer to medical team

14 Paediatric emergencies

Non-Accidental Injury

All staff, medical and nursing, working in an A&E department should be vigilant to the possibility of non-accidental injury. Paediatric opinion and assessment is needed on the slightest suspicion of child abuse.

The **components** of child abuse are:
- Physical injury (non-accidental injury)
- Sexual abuse
- Poisoning or inappropriate drug administration
- Physical neglect
- Emotional deprivation
- Fabricated Illness (Munchausen syndrome by proxy)

The first three of the above are more likely to be seen in an A&E department.

The **possibility** of child abuse may be raised in the presence of the following findings:

HISTORY

Story inconsistent with physical findings
Story incompatible with motor development of child
Inexplicably long delay in presentation
Frequently changing story

PHYSICAL FINDINGS

Bruises
   Of varying ages (different colours)
   With recognizable patterns (e.g. fingers)
Skin lesions
   Bite marks
   Cigarette burns
   Scalds with glove and stocking or grid distribution
Oral lesions
   Frenal tears
   Dental trauma
Limb Injuries
   Spiral fractures
   Lower limb fractures in infants

>

219

    Metaphyseal fractures of long bones
    Calcified subperiosteal haematoma
    Multiple fractures of different ages
Subdural haematoma
Retinal haemorrhages (from forcible shaking)
Visceral rupture

PARENTAL PREDICTORS of CHILD ABUSE, which are of additional help at suspecting child abuse:

Mother
    Young
    Unmarried
Father
    Personality disorder
    Criminal record
    Frequent absences
Both parents
    Social isolation
    Mental illness
    Victims of child abuse themselves

Once child abuse is suspected, prompt referral for further assessment by the paediatric team is indicated. Prior to referral it is often worth checking the local **at risk register** to see if the child is on the at-risk list.

A non-judgemental approach is necessary and the suspicions must not be declared to the parents, who should be informed that a second opinion is being sought for the management of the child's presenting problem(s).

The Crying Baby

The persistently crying infant may occasionally be brought to the A&E department if the parents are finding it difficult to cope. Most of these children require paediatric assessment, not only to detect underlying pathological processes causing crying but to investigate abnormal family dynamics that may be contributory.

The initial **ASSESSMENT** consists of:

- Is the crying of recent onset and unusual for the child?
- Is the character of the cry abnormal?
- Is crying associated with feeding?
  Painful lesions in the mouth
  Nasal obstruction
  Problems with milk delivery (too slow or too fast)

A full **PHYSICAL EXAMINATION** should be carried out.

The Limping Child

ASSESSMENT

Any history of recent trauma
  Trauma may be unwitnessed and hence unreported
Pain
Systemic symptoms: fever, refusal to feed
Prior similar episodes
Does the child look well or ill?
Check temperature
See what happens on attempting to stand up the child
Look at both lower limbs

Look
  Redness
  Bruising
  Joint swelling
  Skin lesions, e.g. puncture marks, abrasions

Feel
  Local warmth
  Tenderness
    Especially over occult tibial fractures in children

Move
  Passive movements of hips, knees, ankles, looking for provocation of pain, restriction of movement and protective muscle spasm

In the absence of convincing trauma, the following are likely possibilities:

Ill child
  Septic arthritis
  Acute osteomyelitis
  Sickle cell disease
  Acute arthritis
  Leukaemia
  Tumour

Well-looking child
  Irritable hip
  Perthes' disease

>

INVESTIGATIONS

Venous blood
FBC, ESR
Blood culture (if toxic)

X-ray of hip
Evidence of Perthes' disease

X-ray of tibia
Suspected toddler's fracture of tibia

Ultrasound of hip
May show joint effusion

MANAGEMENT

Admit if fever
           toxic
           severe protective muscle spasm

Children with irritable hip may be treated on an outpatient basis with daily review

IRRITABLE HIP

Commonly seen in children between the ages of 5 and 10 years

The presenting **features** include:

- Acute or gradual onset of pain in the thigh and knee
- Painful limp, with refusal to bear weight on the involved limb
- History of preceding upper respiratory tract infection or of minor trauma
- Passive movement of the hip reveals restriction of movement with protective spasm
- No systemic symptoms are present

Febrile Convulsions

Febrile convulsions are common and dramatic, proving distressing to parents and other onlookers. They are associated with a rapid rise in body temperature.

Immediate **MANAGEMENT** consists of:

Reduction of body temperature
Remove clothing
Tepid sponging

Rapid stopping of convulsions
Diazepam 0.25 mg/kg slowly intravenously or rectally if intravenous access difficult
Paraldehyde 0.15 mg/kg deep intramuscularly is useful as second-line therapy

PAEDIATRIC REFERRAL

Admission is required in:
- All children with the first fit
- All children aged 18 months or under
- Complex seizures
    Lasting longer than 15 minutes
    Focal features
    Repeated episodes in 24 hours
- Difficult social circumstances

TYPICAL FEATURES OF BENIGN FEBRILE CONVULSIONS

- Usually occur between the ages of 6 months and 5 years
- Generalized tonic–clonic seizures
- Last less than 15 minutes
- Normal neurological examination

For the child who is no longer fitting, document:
- Is this the first or a recurrent episode?
- Is there evidence of infection of
    Throat
    Ears
    Chest
    Urine

>

> **Febrile Convulsions**

- Are there skin rashes?
- Are there signs of meningitis?
    Most children under the age of 18 months require
        diagnostic lumbar puncture
- Family history of febrile convulsion or epilepsy
- Immunization status

Croup (Acute Laryngotracheobronchitis)

This is a clinical syndrome characterized by:

- A harsh barking cough
- Hoarseness of voice
- Inspiratory stridor
- Respiratory distress

which occurs in children aged 6 months to 3 years and usually is preceded by an upper respiratory tract infection.

The symptoms usually occur, or are worse, at night.

ASSESSMENT OF THE DEGREE OF AIRWAY OBSTRUCTION is made by:

- Colour of the child: pink or cyanosed
- Posture of the child
- Sternal and intercostal recession
- Pulse rate
- Ability to swallow

ADMISSION is indicated if there is evidence of:

Airway obstruction at rest, evidenced by subcostal and intercostal recession
Use of accessory muscles of respiration

Inadequate ventilation
Increasing restlessness
          pulse rate
          respiratory rate
Cyanosis
Exhaustion

In a proportion of cases **home management** may be possible, in which case steam inhalation, from a kettle, hot water tap or shower, is useful. Traditionally, a warm moist atmosphere is produced by placing the child in a steam-filled bathroom with the hot water taps running.

Bronchiolitis

Typical **FEATURES**
- Age under 2 years
- Dry cough which is harsh and paroxysmal
- Fever
- Shortness of breath with poor feeding
- Tachypnoea
- Wheezing

Improvement occurs over 5–7 years

The usual **CLINICAL FINDINGS** are of:
- Flaring of the nostrils
- Hyperinflation of the chest
- Suprasternal, intercostal and subcostal recession on inspiration
- Diffuse wheeze and crepitations

Initial **ASSESSMENT** includes:
- Pulse oximetry
- Chest X-ray
    Hyperinflation with flattened diaphragms
    Interstitial pneumonia

MANAGEMENT
Paediatric referral
    Administer humidified oxygen

Acute Epiglottitis

This is an acute life-threatening infection involving the supraglottic structures and nearly always due to *Haemophilus influenzae* type B. It typically affects children aged 2–6 years but can occur at any age.

The presenting **FEATURES** are:

Rapid onset of systemic toxicity with fever and increasing shortness of breath

Associated features include:

- Sore throat
- Dysphagia
- Drooling of saliva
- Inspiratory stridor
- A muffled cry

Once the diagnosis is suspected urgent paediatric, anaesthetic and ENT assistance must be sought.

Do not:

Make the child lie down
Attempt venepuncture
Inject drugs
Attempt to look at the throat
Obtain neck X-rays

Many of the above manoeuvres can help convert partial airway obstruction into complete obstruction.

DEFINITIVE TREATMENT involves:

Transfer to the operating theatre
Induction of general anaesthesia
Direct laryngoscopy to confirm the diagnosis
Oral endotracheal intubation, failing which nasotracheal intubation
An intravenous infusion is set up
Blood is simultaneously taken for culture
Intravenous antibiotics are commenced

15 Ophthalmological emergencies

Red Eye

HISTORY

The following should be checked:

- Trauma, including abrasions to the surface of the globe from fingers, tree branches, etc.
- Use of   welding arc
  hand tools
  power tools
- Use of contact lenses
- Previous eye disease
- Pertinent past medical history, e.g. diabetes mellitus

The nature and duration of **ASSOCIATED SYMPTOMS** must be ascertained:

- Blurred vision
- Reduced visual acuity
- Itching
- Foreign body sensation
- Photophobia
- Discharge, leading to sticking together of eyelids on waking in the morning

On **EXAMINATION**, the following should be looked for:

Eyelids: swelling
  redness
  discharge

Pattern of redness
Conjunctiva: localized
  diffuse
  circumcorneal

Cornea
  Transparency
  Fluorescein staining

Anterior chamber
  Depth
  Pus (hypopyon)
  Blood (hyphaema)

>

> Red Eye

Pupil
   Size
   Shape
   Outline
   Light reaction

Both eyes must be checked

In all cases, visual acuity must be documented using a Snellen Chart

Where vision is grossly impaired, the ability to count fingers or to perceive light must be assessed

Where a slit lamp is available and the user is trained, better delineation of anterior segment problems may be achieved

Based on **HISTORY** and **CLINICAL FINDINGS**, the following categories can be identified:

Painless red eye, usually unilateral
   Spontaneous subconjunctival haemorrhage

Uncomfortable red eye, usually **bilateral** and associated with discharge
   Conjunctivitis
      Lid swelling
      Foreign body sensation
      Discharge
      Sticky eyelids
      Redness of bulbar and palpebral conjunctivae
      Oedema of the conjunctiva (chemosis)

Painful photophobic red eye, usually unilateral
   Corneal abrasion
   Foreign body: corneal/conjunctival
   Dendritic ulcer
      Circumcorneal congestion
      Branching ulcer on fluorescein staining
   Acute anterior uveitis (iridocyclitis)
      Circumcorneal congestion
      Small irregular pupil
      Cloudy anterior chamber

Foreign Bodies in the Eye

These commonly produce acute symptoms leading to A&E attendance.

Initial **ASSESSMENT** includes:

Duration and nature of symptoms, e.g. pain, photophobia
Documentation of visual acuity
A careful look at the surface of the cornea and conjunctiva, which includes eversion of the upper eyelid (as subtarsal foreign bodies are common)
  The cornea is best looked at tangentially, with oblique illumination

Penetrating foreign bodies should be suspected in the presence of a history of:

- Hammering, drilling or grinding metal (particularly without eye protection)
- Glass-induced windscreen injuries
- Blast explosions

In these circumstances X-rays of the orbit and formal ophthalmological assessment is required.

MANAGEMENT

Conjunctival foreign bodies can usually be removed on a cotton bud
Corneal foreign bodies can be removed after instillation of local anaesthetic drops (e.g. benoxinate, amethocaine) into the conjunctival sac
Removal is aided by a sterile 21-gauge needle tip
Fluorescein staining of the cornea after removal is indicated
Residual rust rings are best left in situ and removed after 24 hours
After-care includes instillation of antibiotic ointment in the eye, application of an eye pad and review after 24 hours
Inability to remove a corneal foreign body or lack of training in doing so are indications for ophthalmological referral
All suspected and proven penetrating foreign bodies need ophthalmological assessment

Acute Loss of Vision

Almost invariably ophthalmological assessment is necessary for this presenting symptom. On-site ophthalmic services are not universally available in the UK. Hence careful initial evaluation in the A&E department is necessary to organize appropriate follow-up, which may be organized over the telephone.

Initial **ASSESSMENT** should include answers to the following questions:

- Is it unilateral or bilateral?
- Is pain present?
- Were there any warning symptoms, e.g.
    Floaters
    Light flashes
    Shadows in visual field
- Is there a history of trauma?
- Was any toxin consumed, e.g. methanol
- Is there a relevant past medical history: AIDS, diabetes mellitus

On **EXAMINATION**, the following points should be determined:

Visual acuity in both eyes, using a Snellen Chart
    Use patient's spectacles/contact lenses if a refractive error is present
Colour of the globe: red or white
State of the cornea: clear or hazy
Depth of the anterior chamber
Pupillary light reaction
    Afferent pupillary defect
    Relative afferent pupillary defect
Intraocular pressure on digital palpation
Ophthalmoscopy
    Red reflex in the pupillary area
    Visualization of all four quadrants of the retina, and the macula
    Visual fields by confrontation, using a red pin

>

> Acute Loss of Vision

Based on the history and initial findings, the following categories can be identified:

Red painful eye
Acute angle closure glaucoma
Acute anterior uveitis

White painless eye
1. **Normal fundus**
   Afferent pupillary defect
   Optic neuritis
   Optic nerve compression
   Normal pupillary reactions
   Occipital lobe infarction (cortical blindness)
   Hysteria; malingering (both dangerous diagnoses for the inexperienced)

2. **Abnormal fundus**
   Vitreous haemorrhage
   Retinal detachment
   Central retinal artery occlusion
   Central retinal vein occlusion

White painful eye
Retrobulbar neuritis
Giant cell arteritis with anterior ischaemic optic neuropathy

Trauma to the Eye

Trauma to the eye should be suspected:

- In all cases of blunt trauma producing a black eye (i.e. periorbital haematoma)
- All full-thickness lacerations of the eyelids
- All major facial injuries, including burns
- Blast injuries
- All foreign bodies on the surface of the eye
- All facial injuries leading to altered visual acuity or blurred or double vision

INITIAL ASSESSMENT

In multiple trauma ensure patent airway, adequate breathing and stable circulatory status

Always check visual acuity (using spectacles if patient needs them for refractive error)

Document extraocular movements and visual fields

Look at the eye

If suspected penetrating injury, no further examination in A&E should be carried out. The patient must be kept recumbent, an eye shield taped in place and urgent ophthalmological referral made

Tetanus prophylaxis status should be documented

In suspected blunt trauma, look for:

Subconjunctival haemorrhage and its distribution

Bleeding into the anterior chamber

Pupil size and light reaction

Clarity of the lens

State of the optic fundus

16 Ear, nose and throat emergencies

Epistaxis

IMMEDIATE ASSESSMENT

If bleeding is ongoing, the patient must be instructed to pinch the nostrils and breathe through the mouth

Local ice pack application may be of some help

Vital signs must be documented

If hypotension or tachycardia are present, secure venous access, take venous blood for FBC and grouping and cross-matching, and commence volume replacement.

A rapid **history** must be elicited, concentrating on:

- Duration of bleeding
- Source of bleeding: unilateral or bilateral
- Prior episodes of epistaxis
- Postnasal drip: a sensation of blood trickling down the throat
- History of bleeding diathesis
- Current medication (e.g. anticoagulants)
- Past medical history (e.g. hypertension)

An attempt should be made in the A&E department to determine the source of bleeding. This is particularly important in hospitals with no on-site ENT surgical backup.

This can be achieved by:

- Sitting the patient up and providing a bowl to spit into
- Ensuring a good examination light
- Suction to clear the nostrils of blood clots
- Introduction of a nasal speculum into each nostril successively
- Application of cotton wool pledgets impregnated with topical vasoconstrictor, e.g. adrenaline (1 in 1000), may aid visualization

The most common source of epistaxis is anteriorly from a point on the antero-inferior portion of the nasal septum (Little's or Kiesselbach's area).

If a clear bleeding point is visualized, **chemical cautery** with a moistened silver nitrate stick is often helpful. The >

patient is observed for 1 hour thereafter. No nose blowing or picking for 24 hours is advised.

If an anterior bleeding site is not visualized, or not controllable with the above method, ENT referral is indicated.

For uncontrollable anterior bleeding, bilateral anterior nasal packing with ribbon gauze lubricated with BIPP (Bismuth Iodoform Paraffin Paste) is indicated and can be performed in A&E if trained personnel are available.

For posterior nasal bleeding, Foley catheter balloon tamponade is needed. A lubricated 12 or 14 gauge Foley catheter is introduced through a nostril until the tip presents in the throat. The balloon is then inflated and the catheter pulled back through the nostril until the balloon hitches snugly in the postnasal space. This is useful as a temporizing measure until definitive ENT assessment is possible.

Acute Loss of Hearing

Sudden-onset deafness is a symptom that may often not be accorded the importance it deserves. Almost always, ENT referral is necessary.

HISTORY taking should concentrate on:

- Mode of onset, whether acute or acute on chronic
- Any predisposing features:
    Head injury
    Acoustic trauma (e.g. pneumatic drill, pop concert)
    Ototoxic drugs
    Barotrauma
- Associated vestibular symptoms
    Tinnitus
    Dizziness
- Ear-discharge/bleeding

On **EXAMINATION**, the following should be noted:

Is hearing loss unilateral or bilateral?
The degree of severity of hearing loss
    The ability to hear the ticking of a wrist watch with the
        other ear occluded is a useful screening test
The type of hearing loss: conductive or sensorineural
Presence of spontaneous nystagmus
Otoscopy to visualize the tympanic membrane
    Impacted wax is a common source of acute hearing loss

ENT referral is indicated

Patients with acute sensorineural hearing loss will usually require admission.

Foreign Bodies in the Nose

Usually seen in either children or in adults with learning disability.

The **HISTORY** is that of either:

Witnessed foreign body insertion

or

Purulent, foul-smelling, unilateral nasal discharge, often streaked with blood

TYPES OF FOREIGN BODIES

Vegetable matter

Peas

Corn kernels

Round objects

Beads

Stones

Flat objects

Buttons

Button batteries

MANAGEMENT

Objects clearly visible at the anterior nares may be removed in the A&E department if appropriate instrumentation (nasal speculum, good lighting, bayonet and alligator forceps, and right angle hook) are available

All others should be referred to the ENT department

Button batteries require urgent removal because of the risk of corrosion

Inexpert removal can lead to bleeding from nasal mucosal trauma and to aspiration of the foreign body

Foreign Bodies in the Ear

Metallic

Often round and best removed by ENT surgeons electively

Difficult to grasp with the usual instrumentation available in A&E and traumatic removal carries the risk of damage to the middle ear. Usually blunt right angle hook required

Vegetable matter

Can be removed with alligator forceps

Do not irrigate as this causes swelling by water absorption

Live insect

Drown and kill prior to removal

Cotton wool buds and pieces of paper

Remove with alligator forceps

Acute Dysphagia

INITIAL ASSESSMENT includes:

● Duration of symptoms
● Mode of onset
   Acute: possible impaction of food, dentures
              corrosive ingestion
   Gradually progressive
● Ability to swallow solids
                       liquids
                       saliva

   Asking the patient to drink a glass of water while being
      observed is often informative
● Associated symptoms
   Pain
   Haemoptysis
   Nasal regurgitation of fluids
   Pulmonary symptoms
● Determine possible level of obstruction
   Where does food appear to stick?

HISTORY taking can help delineate the site of the underlying lesion:

Pharyngeal
   Difficulty in initiating swallowing
   Coughing
   Choking
   Nasal regurgitation of fluids
   Sense of obstruction in the throat
Oesophageal
   Sense of obstruction in the chest
   Chest pain on swallowing

MANAGEMENT

Look at throat
Examine neck and chest
Observe process of swallowing
Assess hydration

>

> Acute Dysphagia

X-ray neck and chest if radio-opaque foreign body
impaction likely

Chest X-ray may show oesophageal fluid level in
achalasia

ENT referral is usually required

Medical referral is required if a neurological cause is likely

Gastrografin swallow may be helpful

Acute Dizziness

ASSESSMENT

Duration of symptoms
Is it a hallucination of motion or merely lightheadedness?
Is it continuous or episodic?
Relation to position of head and body
Associated symptoms
  Nausea
  Vomiting
  Sweating
  Fainting
  Tinnitus
  Deafness
History of ear disease
Ototoxic drug ingestion or injection (aminoglycoside antibiotics)

EXAMINATION

As a matter of routine, the following should be checked:
Gait
Coordination
  Straight line walking with eyes open and then closed
  Romberg's test
Hearing
Ears by otoscopy
Cranial nerves
Spontaneous nystagmus
Vital signs
Supine and standing blood pressure

The usual **CAUSES** of acute vertigo include:
With aural symptoms
  Head injury
  Acute labyrinthitis
  Labyrinthine fistula
  Round window rupture
No aural symptoms
  Vasovagal attack
  Vestibular neuronitis

>

VESTIBULAR NEURONITIS

Often seen in A&E departments owing to the dramatic nature of symptoms.

The **features** include:

- Age group 30–40 years
- Acute severe prostrating vertigo and vomiting
- Symptoms aggravated by head movement
- Difficulty in standing up
- No aural symptoms
- Often preceding febrile illness
- Normal otoscopy

MANAGEMENT

Vestibular sedative
   e.g. Stemetil injection
ENT follow-up

17 Infections

Tetanus Prophylaxis

All penetrating wounds are possible portals of entry for tetanus bacilli

Certain wounds are at higher risk of tetanus:

- Wounds contaminated with dirt, soil or faeces
- Crush wounds
- Wounds left untreated for 24 hours or more
- Wounds with retained foreign bodies
- Missile injuries

BASIC IMMUNIZATION consists of:

A course of three spaced doses of tetanus toxoid 0.5 ml intramuscularly

    6 weeks between 1st and 2nd doses

    6 months between 2nd and 3rd doses

MANAGEMENT is based on patient category:

Unimmunized/incompletely Immunized/unknown Immunization status

    Complete course of primary immunization

    Add tetanus immune globulin 250 units if high-risk wound

Immunized (full primary course + booster within 10 years)

    No vaccine needed

Use separate syringes and injection sites for tetanus toxoid and tetanus immune globulin

Substitute diphtheria, pertussis, tetanus (DPT) for tetanus toxoid (TT) in children under 6 years of age, with parental consent

Needlestick Injuries

Prevention is better than managing the injury, which can involve laborious procedures, including documentation, and even a risk of litigation.

PREVENTION

Do not resheath used needles in the absence of specially designed apparatus

Do not pass sharps from hand to hand

Dispose of all needles, knife blades and suture needles in sharps containers, which must not be overfilled

Wear gloves for procedures involving blood, tissue fluid or sharp instruments

Cover cuts and open lesions on the skin with waterproof dressings

Updated hepatitis B immunization

MANAGEMENT OF AN INCIDENT

Wash the wound under a running water tap

Encourage free bleeding by squeezing the area

Donor

Check patient records for hepatitis B/C and HIV status

Take 7 ml blood for testing

Recipient

Take 7 ml blood for serology

Hepatitis B imunoglobulin if needed

Hepatitis B vaccination should be commenced if indicated

If donor is HIV positive, use of AZT prophylaxis should be considered (discuss with virologist)

Organize **follow-up** in hospital occupational health department for hospital staff

Abscesses

An abscess is a localized collection of **pus**

The treatment for an abscess is **incision and drainage**
Antibiotics are not indicated for superficial abscesses of the type that usually present in the A&E department

It is important to recognize **pus under tension** (i.e. persistent severe local throbbing pain worsened on dependency and interfering with sleep)
Adequate incision and drainage requires **adequate anaesthesia**

For small superficial abscesses, **field block anaesthesia** is sufficient

Children and adults with large abscesses require general anaesthesia to allow adequate drainage

Ethyl chloride spray does not provide sufficient anaesthesia to allow unhurried drainage of pus

An abscess must be laid open along its entire extent
The **incisions** should always respect local crease lines
All loculi must be broken down using the finger and all pockets of pus laid open

Packing serves no useful purpose and makes subsequent dressing changes painful

Occasionally the **technique of curettage and primary suture obliteration of the abscess cavity** may be useful

If an abscess is adequately drained, symptoms are rapidly relieved and healing is gratifyingly rapid

Prolonged drainage following incision of an abscess indicates either:

- Inadequate drainage of pus
- Retained foreign bodies
- Infection of the underlying bone with or without sequestrum formation

Hand Infections

These are common in A&E practice.

The basic **ASSESSMENT** consists of:
- Duration of symptoms
- Preceding penetrating trauma
- Systemic symptoms, e.g. fever
- Predisposing illness, e.g. diabetes mellitus
- Sleep disturbance: pus under tension causes persistent throbbing pain worsened by dependency which interferes with sleep
- Evidence of proximal spread of infection
    Lymphangitis
- Treatment prior to coming to A&E

SPECIFIC PRESENTATIONS include:

Paronychia: infection of lateral nail fold resulting in redness, swelling and often subcutaneous and subungual pus

In the presence of pus, incision and drainage is required. Subungual pus usually requires nail plate removal for adequate drainage

Pulp space infection: produces swelling, marked tenderness and induration of the volar pulp of the distal phalangeal segment. Fluctuation is a late sign

Incision and drainage is required under tourniquet control using an incision placed in the natural whorls of the finger

Flexor sheath infection: this is a serious infection causing diffuse finger swelling, associated with a semi-flexed posture of the digit and pain on passive extension. Tenderness extends proximally along the flexor tendon sheath in the palm

The patient must be referred to a hand surgeon for formal incision and drainage

Human Bite Injuries

CAUSES

Clenched fist blow to another person's mouth
Direct bites of finger or hand

SPECIAL FEATURES

High risk of polymicrobial synergistic necrotizing infections, often with unusual organism
Suspect a bite wound with any penetrating wound overlying a metacarpal head

MANAGEMENT

Thorough saline lavage
Do not suture skin
Elevate hand in high sling
Commence antistaphylococcal antibiotic (e.g. Flucloxacillin) and anti-anaerobic agent (e.g. Metronidazole)
Tetanus prophylaxis
Review daily for signs of spreading infection

Fever Following Foreign Travel

The victim of febrile illness following recent foreign travel may attend A&E because of the acuteness of symptoms.

Initial **HISTORY** taking should concentrate on:

Duration of fever
  Countries visited including details of itinerary
  Recreational and other (including sexual) activity while abroad including swimming in inland waters
  Contacts with similar illness
  Insect bites
  Vaccination history
  Antimalarial prophylaxis
  Contact with animals

CLINICAL ASSESSMENT includes:

Documentation of vital signs
Associated symptoms
- Abdominal pain
- Diarrhoea and vomiting
- Pulmonary symptoms
- Skin rash
- Lymphadenopathy

Auscultation of heart and lungs
Abdominal palpation for enlargement of liver and spleen

Initial **INVESTIGATIONS** that may need to be done include:

- FBC
- Urinalysis
- LFT
- Thin and thick blood smears for malarial parasite

Any febrile episode or flu-like illness within the first year (especially within first 3 months) after returning to the UK from a malaria endemic zone must be considered as due to malaria until proven otherwise.

Having had adequate anti-malarial chemoprophylaxis does not exclude the possibility of malaria.

18 Trauma

Major Trauma

The management of major trauma victims should follow the principles laid down in the Advanced Trauma Life Support (ATLS) manual of the American College of Surgeons.

It may not always be easy to identify the patient who has sustained major trauma, especially if initially there is a degree of cardiovascular compensation for covert blood loss.

The following categories of patients should, however, be submitted to a trauma team approach using the ATLS protocol.

1. All trauma victims with impaired conscious level (irrespective of whether alcohol or other drugs are involved)
2. All trauma victims with signs of shock (peripheral vasoconstriction, sweating, tachycardia, hypotension)
3. All trauma victims with clinically apparent multiple long bone fractures
4. All victims subjected to situations highly predictive of high velocity impact

   Free falls from heights of 20 feet or over

   Motor vehicle/motor vehicle or motor vehicle/pedestrian impacts with impact velocity of 20 miles per hour or over

   Motor vehicle accidents in which the victim has been ejected from the vehicle

   Motor vehicle accidents in which another vehicle occupant has died

   Motor vehicle accidents with severe damage to the vehicle

A systematic ordered approach to major trauma is essential to minimize errors of omission and commission and to prevent unnecessary deaths during the golden hour after the incident leading to trauma.

The steps involve:

>

CONFIRMING AND MAINTAINING AIRWAY PATENCY WITH SIMULTANEOUS CONTROL OF THE CERVICAL SPINE

Chin lift or jaw thrust

Keep neck immobile in neutral position at all times (initially by holding the head; subsequently by a combination of semi-rigid collar application, along with taping the forehead to the trolley and placement of sandbags or intravenous bags of fluid on either side of the head)

Open mouth and remove foreign bodies (e.g. dentures, clots) manually and suck secretions (vomitus, blood) with rigid wide bore sucker

Insert oropharyngeal airway

Commence high flow oxygen (10–12 litres per minute) via face mask (use nonrebreathing mask with resevoir bag)

Partial airway obstruction or the likelihood of continued airway soiling by bleeding warrants oral endotracheal intubation by an experienced anaesthetist

Complete upper airway obstruction indicates the need for needle cricothyroidotomy to buy time prior to definitive measures (e.g. tracheostomy)

CHECK ADEQUACY OF BREATHING

Feel for air movement at the mouth and nose

Expose chest and look for chest expansion

Determine respiratory rate

Listen to both sides of the chest for air entry

If a tension pneumothorax is diagnosed, i.e. asymmetrical chest associated with progressive cardio-respiratory failure, immediate decompression via anterior 2nd intercostal space in the midclavicular line is needed

Any open sucking chest wounds should be occluded with gauze pad

Commence continuous SaO_2 monitoring by pulse oximetry

>

ASSESS CIRCULATION AND CONTROL BLEEDING

Check pulse rate, regularity and volume
> peripheral perfusion
> skin colour

Control external bleeding by pressure dressings
> Scalp bleeding may be controlled by full thickness haemostatic sutures

Insert two large bore (14 or 16 gauge) cannulae in the antecubital fossae, and simultaneously withdraw at least 20 ml blood for baseline haematology, biochemistry, and grouping and cross matching of at least 6 units type specific whole blood

If access is difficult, long saphenous or basilic venous cutdowns are indicated

Commence continuous ECG monitoring

Insert urethral catheter and commence hourly urinary output monitoring (not when blood visible at external urethral meatus)

Commence volume replacement with crystalloid solutions

Continued haemodynamic instability at this stage may indicate significant intra-abdominal bleeding warranting laparotomy or significant intrathoracic bleeding warranting chest tube placement

DISABILITY

Determine level of consciousness using the AVPU method
> Alert
> responsive to **verbal** stimulus
> responsive to **painful** stimulus
> **unresponsive**

EXPOSURE

Completely undress patient, cutting off clothes where needed

The above constitute primary survey and resuscitation, which proceed simultaneously. Unexpected deterioration during the course of this protocol should warrant reassessment of the areas previously dealt with.   >

SECONDARY SURVEY

This comprises a head to toe assessment of the patient whose airway is patent, breathing (spontaneous or assisted) adequate and who is haemodynamically stable. This includes the insertion of fingers or tubes in all body orifices.

The following are done in this stage:

Glasgow coma score

Head and **face** examination

Chest

Abdomen

Perineal and rectal exam

Limbs

Back (after log rolling)

X-rays in the A&E department

   Cervical spine (lateral)

   Chest (AP)

   Pelvis (AP)

Limb fractures are splinted

Arrangements are made for specialised radiology where appropriate: e.g.

   CT head scan

   Abdominal ultrasound

   Further views of the cervical spine and limbs

Diagnostic peritoneal lavage may be carried out in the situation where abdominal bleeding is likely

>

> Major Trauma

Primary survey and resuscitation proceed simultaneously.

1. **Airway and cervical spine control**
   Can the patient talk? (this implies a patent airway and intact cerebral function)
   Keep neck in line, immobile in neutral position at all times
   If unresponsive, clear upper airway (manually and by suction) (noisy breathing indicates partial obstruction)

2. **Breathing**
   Is there air movement at the mouth? (feel)
   Expose chest: look at and listen to both sides
   Note respiratory rate
   If not breathing, intubate and ventilate
   Drain tension pneumothorax (clinical diagnosis)
   Attach probe of pulse oximeter

3. **Circulation and haemorrhage control**
   Control external bleeding by pressure dressing/sutures for scalp wounds
   Are peripheral pulses palpable?
   Check blood pressure and heart rate. Institute continuous monitoring
   Two large-bore (14 G) lines – antecubital. Failing this, venous cut-down
   Blood (20 ml) taken), Cross-match
   Blood giving set for fluid administration
   Connect litre bags of fluid
   Pass urinary catheter. Institute hourly collection
   Resuscitative laparotomy

4. **Disability: alert, vocal, responds to stimuli, painful, unresponsive (AVPU)**

5. **Exposure**
   Cut off all clothing

6. **X-rays**
   Lateral cervical spine
   Chest
   Pelvis

>

7. **Secondary survey**
   Glasgow Coma Score
   Head to toe exposure and examination
   Log rolling (four persons)
   Check back
   Tubes and fingers in all orifices
   Abdominal ultrasound/diagnostic ⎫
     peritoneal lavage (US/DPL)   ⎬ if
   CT head scan   ⎪ haemodynamically
   Other X-rays   ⎭ stable
   Splint limb fractures
8. **Definitive treatment**
9. **Transfer**

Soft-Tissue Trauma

Soft tissue injuries should be described using commonly accepted terms, as follows:

1. With intact skin
- Contusion or bruising
- Haematoma
- Degloving injury
- Crush injury

2. With disruption of skin continuity
- Abrasion
- Friction burn
- Puncture or stab wound
- Incised wound
- Laceration
  Linear or simple
  Stellate or complex
  Flap
- Degloving injury
- Burn
- Tissue loss

Various combinations of the above may coexist in a given injury

Where possible, diagrams or even Polaroid photos of complex injuries constitute an indispensable part of the clinical record

Further characterization of a **flap laceration** may include:
- Site
- Shape of flap, e.g.
  Semicircular
  Triangular
  Rectangular
- Length to breadth ratio
- Skin colour:
  pale (ischaemic)
  blue (venous congestion)
- Thickness

Wound Management

Wound management depends on the following wound characteristics:

Site
Age of injury
Mechanism of injury
  Tidy: cut
  Untidy: crush
       shear
       avulsion
Whether clean or contaminated with soil, dirt or faeces
Presence or absence of tissue loss
  Do not be misled by wound edge retraction due to skin
    elasticity
Circumstances of injury
  Accidental
  Suicidal
  Homicidal
Tetanus prophylaxis status
Presence of associated injury to
  Nerves
  Blood vessels
  Tendons
  Bones
  Joints
Possibility of foreign body retention
  Organic: wood, cloth
  Inorganic: metal, glass (X-ray)

GENERAL PRINCIPLES OF WOUND MANAGEMENT

Clean with isotonic saline
To aid cleaning, local or even general anaesthesia may be
  needed
Remove all visible foreign particulate matter
Scrub skin if ingrained dirt is present to prevent tattooing
Excise necrotic fat and muscle
Select appropriate closure technique
  Sutures

>

> Wound Management

Steristrips
Glue (Histoacryl)
Delayed primary closure
Healing by granulation
Skin graft
Flap cover

Do not close primarily wounds that are:

Over 12 hours old (24 hours for face and scalp)
Infected
Contaminated by soil or faeces
Caused by human bites
Accompanied by severe crushing of tissues

Skin Suturing

Select appropriate size and material for region of body
  being sutured

Avoid crushing the skin with heavy toothed forceps

Take equal tissue bites

Take a wider bite of tissue in the depths of the wound
  rather than at the surface

    Enter skin perpendicular to skin edge which is held
  up, with forearm fully pronated

    Follow curve of needle and fully supinate forearm by
  the time the needle is withdrawn

    This produces eversion of the skin edges

Do not tie the sutures tightly

Place sutures equidistant

Give a date for planned suture removal, usually at the
  GP's surgery

RECOMMENDED TIMES FOR SUTURE REMOVAL

Scalp 7 days

Face 4–5 days

Chest wall 10 days

Abdomen 10 days

Back 10–14 days

Upper limbs 7–10 days

Lower limbs
  Proximal 10 days
  Distal 14 days

If prolonged wound support is required, replace sutures
  with steristrips

Prolonged suture retention causes unsightly cross-
  hatching as well as predisposing to sepsis

Consider the use of absorbable skin sutures in certain situations, e.g. hands of children

Never use absorbable sutures on the face

Retained Foreign Bodies

TYPES

Organic (reactive)
  Wood
  Plant, e.g. thorns, spines
  Animal
Inorganic (inert)
  Glass
  Metal

Suspect possibility with any penetrating injury

PRESENTATIONS

Information volunteered by the patient
Delayed resolution after penetrating injury
  Persistent pain
  Persistent swelling
  Sepsis
  Draining sinus
Unexplained soft-tissue lump
  Foreign body granuloma
  Monarticular synovitis

ASSESSMENT

Mechanism of injury
Causative agent
Palpate site
X-rays
  Radio-opaque foreign bodies
    e.g. metal, glass
  Secondary changes
    soft-tissue swelling
    periosteal reaction
    osteolytic lesions

Wood will show on ultrasound or on a CT scan

MANAGEMENT

Removal is not always indicated

>

> Retained Foreign Bodies

Indications for removal:

- Symptomatic: persistent pain
- Reactive: wood, rose, thorn
- Functional restriction: tendon or nerve dysfunction
- Location: subungual
         intra-articular
- Sharp and likely to migrate: needle

Removal is seldom urgent and should only be attempted when appropriate expertise is available. Blind unsupervised exploration in the A&E department is mentioned only to be condemned.

The usual requirements for removal of foreign bodies that are not visible or palpable under the skin include:

- Adequate anaesthesia
- Bloodless field: tourniquet
- Adequate exposure
- Access to portable X-rays or image intensifier for radio-opaque foreign bodies

Major Burns

DEFINITION

Greater than 15% of body surface area involved in adults
Greater than 10% of body surface area involved in children

INITIAL ASSESSMENT

Airway

Check patency
High flow oxygen by face mask
Be aware of high risk of airway obstruction in the presence of smoke inhalation and of massive facial oedema and request anaesthetic assessment
Check breathing
Consider need for chest escharotomy for constricting burns
Check circulatory status
  Peripheral perfusion
  Vital signs
Secure venous access
  14 or 16 gauge cannulae in upper limbs, preferably via unburned tissue
  If necessary, cut down on veins
  The help of a paediatrician facilitates venous cannulation in children
Simultaneously take venous blood for baseline FBC, U&E, group and save
Commence plasma protein fraction. Run in initially, as patient is usually 1 hour behind by this time on fluid losses
Give intravenous analgesia if required
  Morphine 0.2 mg/kg titrated to patient's needs
Consider escharotomy for circumferential or near circumferential burns causing distal limb ischaemia or restriction of chest movement
  This is a bedside procedure, not requiring anaesthesia. Cut through entire length and thickness of eschar in mid-lateral lines of limbs and mid-axillary lines of chest wall. Secure haemostasis thereafter

>

> Major Burns

Assess the extent of the burn using the Rule of Nines for
adults or Lund and Browder charts (Fig. 6) for children

RULE OF NINES

	% Body surface area
Head	9
Right upper limb	9
Left upper limb	9
Right lower limb	18
Left lower limb	18
Anterior trunk	18
Posterior trunk	18
Neck	1

The area of the closed palm of the patient's hand is
roughly 1% of his or her body surface area

Calculate fluid requirements using the Muir and Barclay
(Mount) Vernon Formula, after noting the estimated
time of the burn

Look for other injuries

Fractures of the limbs (e.g. falls from burning buildings
or involvement in automobile accidents)

Burns to the eyes

Pass nasogastric tube if vomiting

Pass urethral catheter and commence hourly urine output
measurement

Tetanus prophylaxis

Refer to Regional Burns Unit

Organize transfer with nursing and anaesthetic accompa-
niment only after adequate fluid replacement is
commenced and airway and breathing stabilized

FLUID REPLACEMENT FORMULA

Mount Vernon Formula

Divide the first 36 hours from time of burn (not time of
arrival in hospital) into six periods of 4, 4, 4, 6, 6 and 12
hours

>

> Major Burns

In each period give plasma aliquot equal to:

$$\frac{\text{Body surface area involved (\% burn)} \times \text{body weight (in kg)}}{2}$$

If plasma protein fraction is used, increase calculated volume by one-third

Adjust formula if urine output not adequate

Basic **DOCUMENTATION** should include:

- Time of burn
- Mechanism of burn
- Likelihood of smoke inhalation
- First aid measures used
- Body weight
- Past medical history
- Allergies
- Tetanus immunization status
- Amount and rate of fluid administration

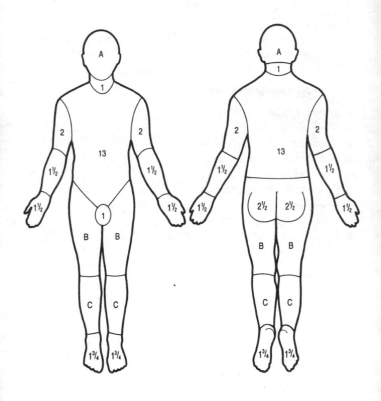

Relative percentage of body surface area
affected by growth

Area	Age 0	1	5
A = ½ of head	9½	8½	6½
B = ½ of one thigh	2¾	3¼	4
C = ½ of one leg	2½	2½	2¾

Ignore
simple erythema

Partial thickness loss
(PTL)
Full thickness loss
(FTL)

Region	%	
	PTL	FTL
Head		
Neck		
Ant. trunk		
Post. trunk		
Right arm		
Left arm		
Buttocks		
Genitalia		
Right leg		
Left leg		
Total burn		

10	15	Adult
$5\frac{1}{2}$	$4\frac{1}{2}$	$3\frac{1}{2}$
$4\frac{1}{2}$	$4\frac{1}{2}$	$4\frac{3}{4}$
3	$3\frac{1}{4}$	$3\frac{1}{2}$

Fig. 6 Lund and Browder charts.

Burns

INDICATIONS FOR ADMISSION
Major burns
Involving over 15% of body surface area in adults and over 10% in children
Circumferential chest and limb burns
Full-thickness burns of critical areas
Fingers
Eyelids
Burns of both hands or both feet
Facial burns with significant swelling
Electrical burns
Non-accidental burns in children

ASSESSMENT OF EXTENT OF BURNS IN ADULTS
Rule of Nines
See table on page 272

BURN WOUND ASSESSMENT
Clues to **depth of burn**
Mechanism of burn
Electrical and flame burns are usually deep
Scalds tend to be superficial or of mixed depth
Temperature of burning agent
Duration of contact with burning agent
Unconsciousness due to seizure or alcohol intoxication may lead to prolonged contact and deep burns
Site of burn
Whether thick skin (e.g. palms, soles, back) or thin skin (e.g. dorsum of hand)
Appearance of burn
Redness: superficial burn
Blistering: dermal burn
Pale and waxy with diminished capillary return or blanching with pressure: deep dermal
Hard, blue, leathery surface with thrombosed veins: full thickness

>

Sensation in burn
  Hyperaesthesia to pin prick (sterile 21-gauge needle):
    superficial
  Analgesic response (reduced sensation): deep dermal
  Anaesthetic to pin prick: full thickness

BURN WOUND MANAGEMENT

Exposure
  Face
  Perineum
  Genitalia
  Buttocks

Dressings
  Limbs
  Torso
  Dressings should be non-adherent, occlusive and
    absorb exudate

Early excision and skin grafting
  Full-thickness burns
  Some deep dermal burns

Polythene bags or gloves with Flamazine cream application
  Extensive hand burns

Blisters
  If large or tense: aspirate
  If septic: deroof

Superficial burns heal in 2–3 weeks and need dressings
  to protect from infection and to absorb exudate
Deep dermal burns heal with excessive scarring in 3–6
  weeks and benefit from early tangential excision
Full-thickness burns need formal excision and grafting
Mixed depth burns require grafting of large areas not
  healed within 3 weeks

Electrical Injuries

DOCUMENT
Type of current: AC or DC
Voltage
Amperage
Duration of contact
Site of contact
History of
   Loss of consciousness
   Associated fall
   Seizures
Need for CPR at the scene or en route
Symptoms of acute onset

MANAGEMENT depends on voltage of the source responsible.

Voltage over 1000 V constitutes high voltage for the purposes of classification

High voltage injuries
Secure venous access
Intravenous fluid replacement must be guided by adequacy of hourly urine output as extent of surface injury does not adequately reflect extent of fluid replacement
12-lead ECG
Continuous ECG monitoring
Venous blood: cardiac enzymes
Look for associated injuries
   Fractures of vertebrae, long bones
Refer to Regional Burns Unit for admission

Low voltage contact burn
Look for entry and exit sites
May need plastic surgery referral for possible primary excision

Head Injury

Head injury forms a significant portion of the workload of an A&E department. The main priority is to identify high-risk patients from the majority, who have minor self-limiting injury. Identification of the seriously ill patient does not usually prove to be a diagnostic challenge.

It is useful to recognize the following syndromes, whose presentation, management and outcome are different:

- Mild closed injury (the majority of A&E attenders)
- Open injury
  Compound vault fracture
  Basal fracture with dural tear
- Intracranial haematoma
- Coma

MINOR CLOSED INJURY

Assessment

Time and mechanism of head injury
Loss of consciousness ('knocked out' is an imprecise term and needs clarification)
Amnesia, including duration of post-traumatic amnesia
Glasgow Coma Score
Scalp bruising/laceration
Pupil size and light reaction
Optic fundi
Discharge from ears/nostrils
History of vomiting
Alcohol consumption
Current medication
Neck symptoms

CRITERIA FOR SKULL X-RAY

- Loss of consciousness
- Neurological signs or symptoms
- Possible penetrating injury
- Difficulty in clinical assessment, provided patient is cooperative, e.g. alcohol intoxication, post-ictal
- Cerebrospinal fluid (CSF) from blood, nose or ears
- Scalp laceration with palpable fracture   >

CRITERIA FOR ADMISSION

Confusion or depressed level of consciousness at time of examination

Skull fracture

Neurological signs

Difficult assessment, e.g. alcohol intoxication, post-ictal

Bleeding disorder with current coagulation abnormality

Significant blow to head with poor social conditions or lack of responsible adult at home (often the overnight stay ward in the A&E department is the most suitable place to admit these patients)

NEUROSURGICAL REFERRAL is indicated for:

- Coma persisting after resuscitation
- Deteriorating level of consciousness
- Progressive focal neurological deficit
- Open injury
  Depressed vault fracture
  Basal skull fracture
- Abnormal CT scan, after liaison with neurosurgeon or after electronic image transmission

RISK OF INTRACRANIAL HAEMATOMA

No skull fracture
Orientated 1:6000
Not orientated 1:120
Skull fracture
Orientated 1:32
Not orientated 1:4

BASAL SKULL FRACTURE

The fracture is difficult to see on conventional skull X-rays

The fracture should be suspected on clinical grounds

The **features** include:

Anterior cranial fossa
Epistaxis
CSF rhinorrhoea

>

> Head Injury

Bilateral periorbital bruising
Bilateral subconjunctival haemorrhage with no posterior limit visible
Injury to cranial nerves I–VI

Middle cranial fossa

Bleeding from ear
CSF otorrhoea
Injury to cranial nerves VII–VIII

Posterior cranial fossa

Suboccipital and retromastoid bruising (Battle's sign)
Injury to cranial nerves IX–XI

GLASGOW COMA SCORE (GCS)

Eye opening (E)

Spontaneous	4
To command (verbal stimuli)	3
To pain	2
Nil	1

Best motor response (M)

Obeys commands	6
Localized pain	5
Normal flexion	4
Abnormal flexion (decorticate rigidity)	3
Abnormal extension (decerebrate rigidity)	2
Nil	1

Best verbal response

Orientated speech	5
Disorientated speech	4
Words only	3
Sounds only	2
Nil	1

>

> Head Injury

Range
3–15

Severe
E1, M5, V2 or less
GCS 8 or less

Moderate
GCS 9–12

Minor
GCS 13–15

Neck Sprains

Neck sprains are common after vehicular collisions, producing acceleration/deceleration stresses on the neck.

The important **FEATURES** include:
- Speed of impact
- Use of seatbelt
- Use of head restraint
- Time of onset of neck symptoms
  Whether immediate or delayed
- Neurological symptoms, e.g. paraesthesiae in the upper limbs (these can also occur with traction lesions of the brachial plexus)
- Prior neck problems

CERVICAL SPINE X-RAYS are indicated with:
- High velocity impact
- Midline neck tenderness
- Reduced neck mobility
- Neurological symptoms or signs
- Pre-existing neck disease

MANAGEMENT
- Rest in soft collar for 48 hours
- Early active neck mobilization
- Non-steroidal anti-inflammatory agents
- Physiotherapy for severe global restriction of neck movement

Penetrating Neck Injury

INITIAL ASSESSMENT

- Check airway patency
- Check adequacy of breathing
- Check circulatory status
- Commence volume replacement if shocked
- Document mechanism of injury

SUBSEQUENTLY

Look for specific findings suggesting injury to specific structures

Vascular trauma

Pulsatile external bleeding
Expanding pulsatile haematoma
Absent carotid pulsation
Systolic or continuous bruits
Focal neurological deficit

Upper airway trauma

Altered or absent voice
Stridor
Subcutaneous emphysema
Haemoptysis

Nerve trauma

Horner syndrome
Hypoglossal palsy (check tongue protrusion)
Spinal accessory nerve palsy (check shoulder shrugging)

Upper digestive tract injury

Dysphagia
Haematemesis

MANAGEMENT

If haemodynamically unstable, immediate surgical referral
If haemodynamically stable, obtain:
Soft-tissue neck X-ray (A/P and lateral) which may show:
Air in the tissues
Foreign bodies
Prevertebral space widening due to retropharyngeal haematoma

>

> Penetrating Neck Injury

Chest X-ray which may show:
Pneumothorax
Superior mediastinal widening
High hemidiaphragm (due to phrenic nerve palsy)
Refer for surgical management

Facial Soft-Tissue Trauma

Check airway patency
Check for injuries elsewhere that take priority
Determine extent of injury
  Tissue loss
  Presence of embedded dirt
Do not shave eyebrows
Use fine suture material (5/0 or 6/0) of synthetic monofilament
Early suture removal (4–5 days)
Align landmarks
  Hairline
  Forehead creases
  Eyebrows
  Vermilion – cutaneous junction
Refer complicated injuries to plastic surgeon or maxillo-facial surgeon
Children may occasionally require general anaesthesia for adequate repair

Maxillofacial Trauma

The **PRIORITIES** in **ASSESSMENT** are to:

- Ensure airway patency
- Check ventilation and circulation
- Be aware of neck trauma possibly coexisting

Subsequent **DOCUMENTATION** includes:

Mechanism of injury
Elucidation of specific symptoms
    Impaired vision
    Double vision
    Altered occlusion
    Numbness of the cheek and upper teeth
    Bleeding from the nose or ears
    Loose or missing teeth

CLINICAL EXAMINATION includes noting:

Site of swelling and tenderness
Deformity of the cheek or nose
Trismus
Occlusion
Eye injury
Extraocular movements
Infraorbital numbness
Visual acuity
Dental injuries must be documented using the dental formula

X-RAY SIGNS suggesting a **MAXILLARY FRACTURE**

Opacification with or without an air–fluid level in the maxillary antrum
    A tear drop opacity suggests an orbital blow-out fracture
Air in the soft tissues

Nasal Fractures

These are the most common facial fracture in A&E departments. They result from direct trauma, as in assaults or fights.

The diagnosis is essentially clinical:

- Nasal bruising and swelling
- Deviation of the bridge
- Depression of the bridge
- Palpable crepitus
- Epistaxis

In all cases the interior of the nose should be inspected with a bright light via a nasal speculum. This may reveal:

Septal deviation

Septal haematoma

Always enquire about prior nasal trauma and deformity
X-rays are not needed for the diagnosis

MANAGEMENT

Arrange follow-up in around 3–4 days in an ENT or Plastic Surgery Clinic

It is helpful if the patient can bring a previous full-face photograph to help assessment of post-traumatic deformity

Septal haematoma requires urgent drainage to prevent septal necrosis and saddle deformity of the nose. ENT referral is indicated

Mandible Fractures

The priorities are to ensure airway patency, adequacy of breathing and adequate circulatory status

Initial **assessment** should look for:

- Localized bruising
- Malocclusion
- Trismus
- Intraoral bleeding: laceration, sublingual haematoma
- Lower lip anaesthesia

Beware of falls onto the chin. In these cases look for bilateral condylar fractures which can coexist

X-RAYS

Orthopantomography is required
Additional views of the temporomandibular joints may be needed to define the condyles

Refer to a maxillofacial surgeon

Penetrating Chest Trauma

INITIAL ASSESSMENT

- Airway patency
- Adequacy of breathing
  Immediate decompression of suspected tension pneumothorax by aspiration of air via anterior 2nd intercostal space in midclavicular line
- Check circulatory status
- Document vital signs
- Pulse oximetry

If **HAEMODYNAMICALLY STABLE**:

Portable chest X-ray
12-lead ECG
Intercostal intubation for
   Pneumothorax
   Haemothorax
   Gunshot wounds

Indications for **THORACOTOMY**

Extensive bleeding: 1500 ml blood obtained at initial tube insertion
Continued bleeding via chest drains: over 100 ml per hour
Pericardial tamponade
Major airway injury
Oesophageal injury
Great vessel injury
Retained knife blade in chest

Indications for **EMERGENCY ROOM THORACOTOMY**

Very limited and high mortality to be expected
Cardiorespiratory arrest on arrival in A&E department
Signs of life in transit
Still warm
Trajectory of wound indicates possible cardiac injury

If **HAEMODYNAMICALLY UNSTABLE**

Immediate surgical referral (to cardiothoracic surgeon if available on site)

Abdominal Trauma

This can often produce subtle signs or cause difficulties in diagnosis, particularly in unconscious, hypotensive or intoxicated patients.

The initial assessment is directed toward airway patency, adequacy of breathing and ventilation, and haemodynamic status.
All vital signs must be documented.

ASSESSMENT of the abdomen includes:

Inspection
Abrasions
Seat belt marks/clothing imprint marks
Penetrating wounds
Distension
Includes looking at the back and perineum and external
genitalia

Palpation
Tenderness
Involuntary muscle guarding
Rebound tenderness

Auscultation
Bowel sounds
Bruits

Digital rectal and pelvic examination
Measurement of abdominal girth is unreliable

Initial **INVESTIGATIONS** include:

Venous blood: FBC, amylase
Urine: dipstick testing for blood
Abdominal ultrasound or diagnostic peritoneal lavage:
Where the patient is haemodynamically stable but abdominal trauma cannot be excluded on clinical grounds due to difficulty in assessment

Indications for **SURGICAL REFERRAL**
All patients with penetrating trauma

>

> Abdominal Trauma

Blunt trauma with
  Signs of peritoneal irritation
  Signs of acute blood loss unaccountable by losses else-
    where
  Difficulty in assessment, e.g. intoxication

Arterial Trauma

The diagnosis of arterial injury can be easily overlooked or delayed, particularly in the absence of brisk external pulsatile haemorrhage.

It should be suspected in the presence of wounds associated with:

- Active pulsatile external haemorrhage
- Large, expanding or pulsatile haematoma
- Palpable bruit/audible thrill
- Loss of distal pulses
- Signs of distal ischaemia
  Pallor
  Paraesthesiae
  Paresis of muscle groups
- Signs of injury to adjacent nerve
- Proximity of a missile or knife to a major artery
    The object may be tamponading the arterial tear and must not be removed in the A&E department. Premature removal may precipitate torrential haemorrhage

MANAGEMENT

Local pressure dressing to control haemorrhage
Venous access: place large-bore intravenous cannula
Venous blood for FBC: grouping and cross-matching
Commence volume replacement
Refer to a vascular surgeon

Regional Analgesia

Techniques of regional analgesia are suitable for A&E use provided adequate practical training in administration is available.

Useful techniques include:

DIGITAL NERVE BLOCK

Plain lignocaine (2.5–3 ml) is injected into the base of the finger to be anaesthetized at either the level of the proximal phalanx or in the hand between the metacarpal heads. The digital neurovascular bundles lie directly under the palmar skin. For procedures involving the dorsum of the finger, an additional subcutaneous injection is made into the dorsal tissues of the finger. At least 5 minutes should be allowed to elapse before embarking on a procedure.

MEDIAN NERVE BLOCK

About 7–10 ml plain lignocaine is injected around the median nerve at the wrist, between the central two tendons (palmaris longus and flexor carpi radialis). This anaesthetizes the radial $3\frac{1}{2}$ digits.

ULNAR NERVE BLOCK

About 7–10 ml plain lignocaine is injected deep to and medial to the most ulnar tendon in the volar aspect of the wrist (flexor carpi ulnaris).

INTRAVENOUS REGIONAL ANALGESIA (BIER'S BLOCK)

This procedure is very useful for manipulation of fractures of the distal radius. The procedure must be treated in similar fashion to a general anaesthetic and is not suitable for single operator use, i.e. there must be one doctor (preferably with anaesthetic training) to administer the block, and another to carry out the manipulation.

The patient must be starved at least 4 hours before the procedure.

>

> Regional Analgesia

Initial assessment includes determining suitability for the procedure. Intravenous regional analgesia is contraindicated for:

- Children under the age of 12 years
- Patients with sickle cell disease
- Patients with peripheral vascular disease affecting the upper extremities
- Patients with local sepsis

Informed consent is necessary.
Prior to the procedure, the following observations are required:

- Blood pressure
- Weight

Venous access must be obtained both in the limb to be anaesthetized as well as in the opposite upper limb.
ECG and pulse oximetric monitoring must be commenced.
0.5% prilocaine (Citanest) is used for the anaesthetic: usually 35 ml is required for the average 70 kg adult.
The tourniquet to be used should be tested, ensuring there are no leaks in the tubing.
The limb is elevated for exsanguination.
The cuff pressure is taken to about 60 mmHg above systolic blood pressure. This pressure must be maintained for at least 20 minutes after completion of injection of the anaesthetic agent.
The patient should be warned about the typical mottled discoloration of the limb that follows.
At least 10 minutes should be allowed for the anaesthetic to take effect.
The technique is not suitable for procedures lasting over 45 minutes.
The patient should be kept under observation for at least 1 hour after the procedure is completed.

X-Ray Diagnosis of Skeletal Trauma

Examine bone and joints in at least two planes at right angles to each other: A/P and lateral views are usual. Additional oblique views may be needed as well.

Look at the entire length of both bones in fractures of paired bones.

1. Look for signs of fracture
    Fracture line
        Lucent
        Dense (overlap of fragments)
    Step in or bulge in cortex
    Interruption of bony trabeculae (impacted fracture)

2. Look for indirect signs of fracture
    Joint effusion
        Fat pad sign
    Air in joint or surrounding tissues
    Fat–fluid levels

3. Consider the need for
    Special views (e.g. scaphoid, calcaneus)
    Serial examinations
    Comparison films (epiphyseal injuries of the elbow)
    Tomograms

In these situations discussion with an A&E senior doctor or a radiologist is often indicated.

Be aware of the pitfalls in interpretation
- Nutrient canals
- Secondary ossification centres
- Partial epiphyseal fusion

Always correlate abnormal findings with the site of pain and tenderness

Salter-Harris Classification of Epiphyseal Plate Injuries

This useful classification helps give an objective description of epiphyseal injuries, particularly over the telephone, and should be more widely used in A&E departments than it is at present.

There are five injury patterns. The first two types are relatively benign, while types III–V can produce growth disturbance secondary to premature epiphyseal fusion.

TYPES

I   Complete separation of the epiphysis
    No fracture of the bone
II Fracture separation
    Line of separation extends along epiphyseal plate to a variable distance and then through a portion of the metaphysis, leading to a triangular-shaped metaphyseal fragment
III Intra-articular fracture extending from joint surface to deep zone of epiphyseal plate and then along the plate to the periphery
IV Intra-articular fracture extending from joint surface through epiphysis, across entire thickness of epiphyseal plate and through a portion of the metaphysis
V   Severe crushing force applied through epiphysis to one area of the epiphyseal plate

Fractures/Dislocations of the Upper Limbs

FRACTURES OF THE CLAVICLE

Check for
  Neurovascular complications in the upper limb
  Viability of overlying skin
If there are no neurovascular complications and the overlying skin is not at risk of necrosis:

- Collar and cuff sling under clothes
- Follow-up in Fracture Clinic.

If the above complications are present, refer as open reduction and internal fixation may be needed

STERNOCLAVICULAR JOINT DISLOCATIONS

Anterior
  This is a clinical diagnosis, with increased prominence of the medial end of the clavicle
  X-rays are difficult to interpret
  Maintenance of reduction is difficult
  Hence, no attempt at reduction is made; a triangular sling is provided to rest the upper limb, and Fracture Clinic follow-up is arranged

Posterior
  Refer to orthopaedics team for urgent reduction
  May compromise great vessels and trachea

ACROMIOCLAVICULAR JOINT INJURIES

Sprains and subluxations
  Rest in triangular sling for upper limb

Fracture Clinic follow-up

Dislocations
  Cause step at acromioclavicular joint due to increased prominence of lateral end of clavicle
  Refer to orthopaedics team as some surgeons treat with open reduction and internal fixation, especially in young athletic males. If the policy is non-operative, rest the upper limb in a triangular sling and refer to the Fracture Clinic   >

Radiographic visualization may be improved by asking for stress views of the acromioclavicular joints, taken with the patient holding a weight in the hand on the involved side to accentuate the deformity

SHOULDER DISLOCATIONS
Anterior
Cause characteristic deformity with flattening of deltoid contour and a square appearance to the shoulder

An empty space can be felt under the acromion process

Always check distal neurovascular function, including:
Sensation over deltoid (axillary nerve)
Radial pulse
Sensation and power in hand and wrist

Always obtain an X-ray before reduction as fractures may coexist

MANAGEMENT
Nerve or vascular injury (apart from axillary nerve)
Refer to orthopaedics team

Associated fracture
Fracture of neck of humerus
Refer to orthopaedics team
Fracture of greater tuberosity of humerus
Attempt reduction in A&E

No fracture
Attempt reduction in A&E
Use IV midazolam and IV fentanyl or pethidine
Monitor pulse, blood pressure and pulse oximetry
Perform procedure in area with full resuscitation facilities
Warn the patient that if the procedure fails, general anaesthesia will be needed
Post-reduction
Check X-rays
Check neurovascular status
Triangular sling under clothes; a body stocking may in addition be used in young muscular individuals
Follow-up in Fracture Clinic   >

Recurrent Dislocation

Reduction sometimes easier

Rest in sling for 2–3 days thereafter

Fracture Clinic follow-up may not be needed if the patient is already under orthopaedic follow-up

FRACTURES OF THE HUMERAL SHAFT

Assessment

Check elbow and shoulder joints and remainder of upper limb

Check radial nerve function (look for wrist drop)

Check radial pulse and circulation to fingers

Management

Undisplaced or minimally displaced

Collar and cuff sling or U-slab plus collar and cuff sling

Fracture Clinic follow-up

Displaced, or segmental, or with distal neurovascular deficit

Orthopaedic referral

SUPRACONDYLAR FRACTURE OF THE HUMERUS

Check distal neurovascular function

Undisplaced

Collar and cuff sling or posterior above-elbow plaster of Paris (POP) back slab

Fracture Clinic follow-up

Displaced, or with distal ischaemia

Refer to orthopaedics team

Angular and rotary deformity and severe displacements need reduction

POSTERIOR DISLOCATION OF THE ELBOW

Produces a typical deformity with prominent oleocranon and taut triceps tendon, disturbing the normal equilateral triangle formed by the oleocranon and the medial and lateral epicondyles

Check distal neurovascular function

Always obtain an X-ray before reduction as fracture may coexist

> Fractures/Dislocations of the Upper Limbs

No fracture

Attempt reduction in A&E using IV analgesia and sedation

If this fails, refer to orthopaedics team for reduction under
   general anaesthesia

After reduction

   Posterior above-elbow POP back slab and collar and
      cuff sling

   Or collar and cuff sling alone

   Check distal neurovascular function

   Fracture Clinic follow-up

Associated fracture

Refer to orthopaedics team

FRACTURE OF THE LATERAL CONDYLE OF THE HUMERUS

Undisplaced

Collar and cuff sling

Fracture Clinic follow-up

Displaced

Usually a Salter type IV epiphyseal injury, where the actual
   displacement is much more than is readily discerned
   on X-ray.

Refer to orthopaedics team for open reduction and internal
   fixation

FRACTURE OF THE RADIAL HEAD

Check

   Distal neurovascular function

   Elbow extension

   Distal end of ulna for subluxation

Undisplaced

Triangular sling

Fracture Clinic follow-up

Occasionally a large elbow haemarthrosis may need aspiration under aseptic conditions

>

Comminuted, severely displaced or angulated
Refer to orthopaedics team
Some injuries may require radial head excision

FRACTURES OF THE OLECRANON

Undisplaced
Above-elbow posterior POP slab with elbow in 90° flexion
Fracture Clinic follow-up

Displaced
Refer to orthopaedics team for open reduction and internal
fixation

FRACTURES OF THE RADIUS AND ULNA

Check distal neurovascular function

Undisplaced
Above-elbow posterior POP slab
Fracture Clinic follow-up

Displaced or angulated
Refer to orthopaedics team

ISOLATED FRACTURE OF THE ULNA

Always look at the radial head for dislocation: normally a
line passing through the radial head passes through the
humeral capitellum in all projections

No dislocation of radial head
  Undisplaced or minimally displaced
    Above-elbow posterior POP slab
  Displacement moderate to severe
    Refer for possible open reduction and internal fixa-
      tion
Dislocated radial head (Monteggia lesion)
  Refer to orthopaedics team

ISOLATED FRACTURE OF THE RADIAL SHAFT

Always look at the ulna head for subluxation

**Ulnar head subluxation or dislocation (Galeazzi
lesion)**
  Refer to orthopaedics team   >

No ulnar head injury
   Undisplaced
      Above-elbow posterior POP slab
      Fracture Clinic follow-up
   Displaced
      Refer to orthopaedics team

DISTAL RADIAL FRACTURES

These constitute a common form of fracture seen in A&E
   departments

They can be categorized as:

1. With **dorsal displacement of distal fragment**
   Colles' fracture
2. With **volar displacement of distal fragment**
   Smith's fracture
3. **Styloid fractures**
   Radius
   Ulna
4. **Articular rim fractures** (Barton's fracture)

FRACTURE-SEPARATION OF THE DISTAL RADIAL EPIPHYSIS

This is the childhood equivalent of the adult Colles' fracture

Salter type II injury

Reduction under general anaesthesia is usually required

COLLES' FRACTURE

This is a common fracture usually presenting with a typical
   dinnerfork deformity

The distal radial fragment is usually impacted, dorsally and
   radially angulated and dorsally and radially displaced

Always check median nerve function (sensation in the
   radial 3½ digits) and extension of the thumb extensor
   pollicis longus (EPL)

An ulnar styloid fracture may coexist

Reduction is required in all instances except for minor
   degrees of impaction and dorsal displacement only   >

> Fractures/Dislocations of the Upper Limbs

This can be achieved in A&E by either haematoma block, intravenous regional analgesia or axillary block
A below-elbow POP back slab (properly a dorsoradial slab) should be applied thereafter

SMITH'S FRACTURE

This can also be reduced in A&E using one of the above methods. An above-elbow POP back slab is applied with the forearm supinated

COMMINUTED DISTAL RADIAL FRACTURES

These usually follow high-velocity impact in young adults
Orthopaedic referral is required as they are unstable

Fractures/Dislocations of the Lower Limbs

PELVIC FRACTURES

Always check vital signs
  Urine: ability to void and presence or absence of blood
  Neurovascular function in lower limbs
  Abdomen

STABLE FRACTURES: HAEMODYNAMICALLY UNSTABLE

Bed rest
Either in hospital or at home
Fracture Clinic follow-up if sent home
Elderly may need admission on social grounds

UNSTABLE FRACTURE or HAEMODYNAMIC INSTABILITY due to ACTIVE BLEEDING

Refer to orthopaedics team
Bleeding can usually be controlled by external fixation of
  the pelvis

HIP DISLOCATIONS

Posterior

Lower limb held flexed, adducted and internally rotated
Check sciatic nerve function (foot drop)
Check for associated femoral shaft fracture (obtain X-rays
  of entire length of femur)
Refer to orthopaedics team

Anterior

Lower limb held abducted and externally rotated
Check distal pulses as femoral artery can be compressed
Check femoral nerve (quadriceps)
Refer to orthopaedics team

>

SLIPPED CAPITAL FEMORAL EPIPHYSIS

Typically occurs in overweight adolescents
Presets with hip and thigh pain and referred pain in knee
Occasionally pain in knee predominates; in all knee pain
   of uncertain origin the hips should be examined
Painful limp usual
A clear history of acute trauma is not always present
The affected hip demonstrates loss of internal reduction
   and abduction
With passive hip flexion the thigh rotates externally
The injury is a Salter type I injury
Refer to orthopaedics team

X-RAYS

A/P view: a line drawn along the lateral border of the
   femoral neck fails to intersect capital femoral epiphysis
Lateral view: medial and posterior slippage of the capital
   femoral epiphysis

FRACTURE OF SHAFT OF FEMUR

Always
   Check distal neurovascular function
   Check vital signs
   Secure venous access and obtain venous blood for FBC
      and grouping and cross-matching
   Give intravenous analgesia
   Splint before moving for X-rays (Thomas' splint)
   Obtain X-rays including the pelvis (dislocated hip may
      coexist)

Consider analgesia with femoral nerve block
Refer to orthopaedics team
In children consider the possibility of non-accidental
   trauma

>

FRACTURES OF THE PATELLA
Undisplaced
Aspirate tense haemarthrosis of the knee
Undisplaced
POP cylinder
Fracture Clinic follow-up

Displaced: comminuted
Refer to orthopaedics team
May need internal fixation or patellectomy

FRACTURES OF THE TIBIAL CONDYLE
Undisplaced
Aspirate tense haemarthrosis of the knee
POP cylinder
Fracture Clinic follow-up

Depressed
Refer to orthopaedics team

RUPTURED QUADRICEPS TENDON

Typically seen in the middle-aged
Palpable gap in quadriceps tendon
Unable to raise straight leg off couch
Refer to orthopaedics team

ACUTE LATERAL DISLOCATION OF PATELLA

Obtain X rays
Sometimes gets reduced while in X-ray department
Attempt reduction in A&E using IV analgesia and sedation
Thereafter
   POP cylinder or Robert Jones bandage
   Check X-ray
   Fracture Clinic follow-up
If reduction fails, refer to orthopaedics team

>

FRACTURES OF THE TIBIA

Check distal neurovascular function

Compound fractures are relatively common because of the thin adherent overlying skin

Undisplaced and closed

Above-knee POP back slab with knee in slight flexion

Fracture Clinic follow-up

If gross swelling, refer to orthopaedics team because of risk of compartment syndrome

Displaced and compound

Refer to orthopaedics team

FRACTURES OF THE FIBULA

Neck

Check lateral popliteal nerve function (foot drop)

Long leg elastic compression bandage

Stick or crutches to aid ambulation

Fracture Clinic follow-up

Shaft

Long leg elastic compression bandage

Fracture Clinic follow-up

ANKLE FRACTURES – DISLOCATIONS

Check skin viability

Reduce using IV analgesia and sedation and place in well-padded below-knee posterior POP slab before obtaining X-rays

Refer thereafter to orthopaedics team

FRACTURES OF MEDIAL MALLEOLUS

Undisplaced

Below-knee POP back slab and crutches

Fracture Clinic follow-up

Displaced

Refer to orthopaedics team

>

> Fractures/Dislocations of the Lower Limbs

FRACTURES OF LATERAL MALLEOLUS

Undisplaced
Below-knee POP back slab and crutches
Fracture Clinic follow-up

Displaced; usually with **lateral shift of talus**
Refer to orthopaedics team

BIMALLEOLAR AND TRIMALLEOLAR FRACTURES

Refer to orthopaedics team

DIASTASIS OF TIBIOFIBULAR JOINT

Check proximal fibula for fracture
Refer to orthopaedics team

CALCANEAL FRACTURES

Check
  Opposite calcaneus
  Spine for associated injury
Bilateral
Refer to orthopaedics team
Unilateral

  Undisplaced
    Wool and crepe bandage and crutches
    Fracture Clinic follow-up

  Displaced; subtalar angle disrupted
    Refer to orthopaedics team

  Avulsion fractures of Achilles tendon
    Refer to orthopaedics team

TALAR FRACTURES

Undisplaced
Below-knee posterior POP slab and crutches
Fracture Clinic follow-up

Displaced
Refer to orthopaedics team

TARSAL DISLOCATIONS

Refer to orthopaedics team   >

METATARSAL FRACTURES
Shaft
Isolated
Undisplaced
Walking
Below-knee elastic bandage
Fracture Clinic follow-up
Unable to bear weight
Below-knee posterior POP slab and crutches
Fracture Clinic follow-up
Multiple, usually displaced
Refer to orthopaedics team

Base, usually 5th metatarsal
Below-knee POP back slab and crutches and Fracture Clinic follow-up. If walking, below-knee elastic bandage may suffice

TOE INJURIES
X-ray only if deformed
Otherwise X-ray unnecessary and neighbour strapping of toes for symptomatic relief will suffice
If deformed, obtain A/P and lateral X-rays of the involved toe, not of the entire foot
Reduce fractures and dislocations using digital block anaesthesia
Strap adjacent toes
Check X-rays
Fracture Clinic follow-up
Also trephine painful subungual haematomas

Spinal Trauma

Should be suspected in the following circumstances:

    Any trauma victim who is unconscious or has an altered level of consciousness

    Post-traumatic pain in the neck or back

    Severe facial trauma

    Neurological symptoms and signs in the lower limbs or upper limbs

    Urinary retention

    Priapism

    Refractory hypotension with adequate peripheral perfusion

HIGH-RISK SITUATIONS FOR CERVICAL SPINE TRAUMA

- High-velocity motor vehicle and pedestrian/vehicle accidents
- Falls from a height
- Diving into water
- Sports, e.g. rugby
- Head injury with loss of consciousness

IN THE PRESENCE OF SUSPECTED SPINAL TRAUMA

Move head, torso and lower limbs as a unit

Immobilize the neck with

    Semirigid collar

    Sandbags/intravenous infusion bags on either side

    Forehead taping to the trolley sides

Treat the patient according to ATLS protocols

Determine the upper limit of and extent of neurological dysfunction (motor, sensory and reflex levels)

Obtain X-rays under conditions of medical supervision

With all spinal trauma the following questions need to be answered:

    Is the airway patent, breathing adequate and circulatory status stable?

    Are there any injuries elsewhere?

>

> Spinal Trauma

Are there any neurological symptoms or signs?

If so, what is the upper level of motor, sensory and reflex loss?

Is the injury stable or potentially unstable?

RADIOLOGICAL ASSESSMENT OF THE CERVICAL SPINE

Basic principles

Visualize all seven cervical vertebrae and the C7/D1 junction

Check the alignment by tracing the following lines:

Anterior border of vertebral bodies

Posterior border of vertebral bodies

Spinolaminar line (connecting posterior junction of lamina and spinous processes)

Tips of the spinous processes

Check the prevertebral soft tissues

Vertebral bodies

Disc spaces

Facet joints

Spinal canal (posterior border of vertebral body to spinolaminar line)

Spinous processes

Inspect the odontoid on open mouth views

Instability can be predicted on the following findings:

Widening of the space between spinous processes (fanning)

Facet joint overriding or widening

Fracture with compression of more than 25% of height of vertebral body

Over 3.5 mm anterior vertebral body displacement in relation to an adjacent vertebral body

Over 10° angulation between vertebral bodies

All dislocations

Tear drop fracture of anteroinferior margin of vertebral body

Jefferson's bursting fracture of atlas

Hangman's fracture

Shoulder Injuries

ASSESSMENT
History
Mechanism of injury: how, where, when?
Specific symptoms
    Pain
    Stiffness
    Swelling
    Tenderness (inability to lie on affected side)

CLINICAL EXAMINATION
Expose chest and both shoulders
Look for
    Deformity
        Altered shoulder contour
        Step at acromioclavicular joint
    Swelling
    Muscle wasting
        Supraspinatus
        Infraspinatus
Feel for
    Localized tenderness
    Swelling
    Axillary nerve sensation (lateral arm)
    Distal
        Radial pulse
        Sensation in forearm and hand
        Grip strength in hand
Move
    Abduction and adduction
        Internal and external rotation
    Look for a painful arc in mid range of abduction

Elbow Injury

ASSESSMENT

History
Mechanism: how, where, when?
Specific symptoms
Pain
Swelling
Stiffness

CLINICAL EXAMINATION

Always compare both elbows

Look for
Deformity
Swelling
Skin changes (e.g. redness)

Feel for
Localized tenderness
Local warmth
Swelling
Distally
Radial pulse
Finger sensation

Move
Elbow flexion and extension
Forearm supination and forearm
Wrist flexion and extension
Lack of full elbow extension is a useful marker of significant elbow injury

X-RAYS

Fracture
Effusion: posterior fat pad sign
Should prompt to look for a fracture
If none seen, collar and cuff sling and review in 10 days and possibly X-ray again

PULLED ELBOW

Occurs in children under the age of 4 years

>

> Elbow Injury

Caused by longitudinal traction on the wrist with the elbow
    extended and the forearm pronated (usually by lifting
    the child up by the wrists)
Refusal to use the involved upper limb (pseudoparalysis)
Elbow held extended and forearm pronated
X-rays not necessarily useful and are usually normal
Manipulation is curative
    Flex elbow
    Supinate forearm with pressure on radial head simul-
      taneously
    A palpable click confirms reduction
No after-treatment is usually required
The child can be discharged home with instructions to be
    reviewed in A&E if normal use not regained by the next
    day

Knee Injury

The knee is the largest and most complex joint in the human body. Injury is a frequent cause for A&E attendance. The aim of A&E assessment is to identify significant injuries requiring hospital treatment and follow-up and those that are self-limiting and can be managed in the community.

Assessment begins with the **HISTORY**

Mechanism of injury
  Direct trauma, e.g. blow to or fall onto the knee
  Indirect trauma, e.g. twisting, lateral (valgus) or medial (varus) stress
Where and when did the injury occur?
What was the function of the leg immediately after the injury?
  Was the person able to continue walking running or whatever else was being done at the time?
Specific symptoms
  Pain, including site
  Swelling, if so whether:
    Rapid onset (within 1–2 hours): indicating active bleeding into the joint
    Delayed onset (over 24 hours): indicating reactive exudation of synovial fluid into the joint cavity
  Locking: care must be taken to define precisely this complaint, which may be used uncritically by the general public. Locking refers to the loss of the terminal 5–10° of knee extension due to a mechanical block as opposed to mere pain
Prior knee problems
  Symptoms
  Arthroscopy
  Surgery

EXAMINATION

Examination of the acutely injured knee may be hampered by pain and swelling

>

> Knee Injury

Evaluation of the acutely injured knee should concentrate on:

Inspection
Deformity, e.g. lateral dislocation of the patella
Swelling: whether localized or generalized

Palpation
Localization of tenderness, e.g.
Joint line
Medial or lateral ligaments
Effusion in the joint space

Mobility
Flexion
Extension
Inability to actively extend the knee, as in raising the straight leg off the couch, indicates disruption of the extensor mechanism or a severe injury with haemarthrosis and possible fracture
Lack of terminal 5–10° of extension as compared with the normal knee indicates locking

Stability
Usually stability testing of the acutely painful knee is uninformative

Distal neurovascular function

In knee pain, particularly in adolescents and in the elderly with no abnormality in the knee on examination, the hip joint must be examined as this may be due to referred pain to the knee.

The following categories of knee injury warrant examination and orthopaedic follow-up:

- All fractures
- Haemarthrosis: with or without fracture
  Aseptic aspiration of blood in the A&E department achieves the following:
  Relief of pain
  Reduction of risk of chemical synovitis and adhesions
  Easier examination of the joint   >

> Knee Injury

- Patella dislocations after reduction
- Locked knees
- Ligament injuries with obvious instability
- Possible meniscal injuries

Ankle Injuries

Ankle sprains comprise one of the most common injuries seen in an A&E department.

The basic **ASSESSMENT** consists of:

- Mechanism of injury
    Inversion
    Plantarflexion
    Dorsiflexion
    Direct impact
- Ability to bear weight after the injury
- Nature and site of symptoms
    Pain
    Swelling
- Prior ankle problems

EXAMINATION consists of looking for:

Deformity
    Deformity due to a fracture dislocation requires imme-
        diate reduction in A&E using intravenous analgesia
        and POP back slab application before X-rays, to
        prevent pressure necrosis of the skin
Swelling/bruising, including site
Gait, if able to bear weight

PALPATION

In early injuries it should be possible to localize tender-
    ness to either lateral or medial malleolus or to the
    ligaments
As a matter of routine the foot should be palpated, partic-
    ularly the calcaneus, anterior talus and the 5th
    metatarsal base
Any tenderness in the region of the Achilles tendon
    warrants looking for discontinuity of the tendon
Failure of passive ankle plantarflexion on calf muscle
    squeezing indicates disruption of the tendon

X-RAYS are indicated if:

- There is inability to bear weight

>

> Ankle Injuries

- Gross swelling and bruising
- Localized bony tenderness

and must be considered if the patient is aged over 60 years because of the higher likelihood of a fracture.

Combined X-rays of the ankle and foot are seldom necessary and are usually wasteful of resources.

RUPTURE OF THE ACHILLES TENDON

This injury is often missed, making treatment difficult when eventually diagnosed.

Features

Sudden onset of acute ankle pain often thought to be caused by something hitting the back of the leg, while actively using the limb

Inability to run

Inability to walk on toes leading to a flat-footed gait

Examination

Palpable gap in tendon

Weak plantar flexion of ankle

Failure of passive ankle plantarflexion on calf squeeze with patient prone, e.g. kneeling on both knees on a chair

Management

Orthopaedic referral

Fresh ruptures can be treated by either:

Immediate surgical repair

or by application of a long-leg POP cast with the ankle maximally plantarflexed (equinus)

Delayed diagnosis of ruptures

Surgical repair is indicated

Pretibial Injuries

FEATURES
- Majority are due to blunt trauma
- Three-quarters occur in women over the age of 50 years
- The skin is thin, inelastic and lacks subcutaneous tissue padding
- Steroid therapy may aggravate the injury
- Ischaemia of the lower limb may delay healing (always palpate the dorsalis pedis and posterior tibial pulses)

PRESENTATIONS
Early
    Flap lacerations
    Haematomas
Late
    Skin necrosis
    Cellulitis
    Chronic ulceration

MANAGEMENT
Suturing is not recommended as the thin friable skin often necroses

If **skin viable**
    Unfurl skin edges
    Appose skin edges with Steristrips
    Dress
    Refer for follow-up by the district nurse

If **skin non-viable**
    Obtain plastic surgical opinion
    May benefit from meshed skin graft application and early ambulation

19 Miscellaneous

Acute Problems in Sickle Cell Disease

A variety of acute problems may complicate sickle cell disease, usually producing severe symptoms leading to A&E attendance.

These include:

PAINFUL VASO-OCCLUSIVE CRISES (commonest)

These account for over 90% of emergency admissions in sickle cell disease

Typically acute severe limb pain is produced by small vessel occlusion causing infarction. Chest and abdominal pain can also occur. The haemoglobin level usually remains stable

SEQUESTRATION SYNDROME

This is characterized by acute enlargement of a visceral organ such as the liver or spleen caused by massive sequestration of red blood cells, accompanied by loss of function. Severe systemic upset is present

The haemoglobin level falls while the reticulocyte count is high

Alternatively, girdle syndromes leading to a diffusely tender distended abdomen with paralytic ileus can occur mimicking a surgical acute abdomen

The sickle chest syndrome is associated with shortness of breath, pleuritic chest pain and signs of consolidation

APLASTIC CRISIS

Associated with a fall in haemoglobin level and a low reticulocyte count

HAEMOLYTIC CRISIS

Associated with a fall in haemoglobin and a high reticulocyte count

PRIAPISM
CNS COMPLICATIONS
Stroke

>

EYE COMPLICATIONS
Vitreous haemorrhage
Retinal detachment

MANAGEMENT OF SICKLE CRISIS

Provide adequate **opiate analgesia** on arrival
Morphine 10 mg or diamorphine 10 mg intramuscularly
Commence **rehydration** with intravenous fluids
Children 80 ml/kg body weight/24 hours
Adults   1 litre normal saline over 3 hours
Then 70 ml/kg body weight/24 hours

Oxygen (60%) by mask only if pao_2 less than 10 kPa on air

Consider **broad-spectrum antibiotics**

Obtain **venous blood** for FBC, reticulocyte count, group and save, and culture if sepsis suspected

Refer to on-call medical team or to clinical haematologist where available for admission

Anaphylaxis

This is a life-threatening consequence of a type I hyper-sensitivity reaction, characterized by:

Skin and mucosae
Diffuse itching
Generalized urticaria
Swelling of eyelids, tongue, lips, ears and hands and feet

Respiratory system
Shortness of breath
Tightness in the chest
Wheezing
Hoarseness
Stridor

Cardiovascular system
Hypotension
Tachycardia

The usual **CAUSES** are:

Injectants
Insect bites
Vaccines
Blood products

Ingestants
Food (e.g. peanuts)
Drugs

MANAGEMENT consists of:

Adrenaline 0.5–1.0 ml of 1:1000 (1 mg in 1 ml) subcu-taneously or intramuscularly
Slow intravenous administration with ECG monitoring is indicated if the patient is shocked

Antihistaminics
Chlorpheniramine 5–10 mg intravenously or intramus-cularly

Steroids
Hydrocortisone 100–200 mg intravenously or intramus-cularly   >

> Anaphylaxis

Plasma expanders must be used for persisting hypotension

Medical referral is indicated for observation, continuing treatment and follow-up

The Homeless

Because of the open access no-appointment system of provision of care in A&E departments, the homeless may use A&E departments for both primary and secondary health care, as well as for access to social services.

A sympathetic non-judgemental approach is needed in dealing with the homeless, who form a small but significant part of the workload of inner city departments.

SPECIFIC PROBLEMS OF THE HOMELESS include:

Alcohol abuse
Drug abuse
Vulnerability to violence and sexual abuse
Parasitic infestations, e.g. lice
Poor oral hygiene, with dental problems
Leg ulcers
Mental illness
Tuberculosis
Malnutrition
Hypothermia

IMPORTANT ASPECTS of MANAGEMENT include:

Effective liaison with **Social Services**
Awareness of relevant statutory and voluntary agencies in the locality
Prior records of A&E attendance and clinical records thereof
Awareness of GPs willing to register and follow-up the homeless